To J.W.
I know you
miss her...

Schafer

In Loving Memory Of
Marianne Schafer

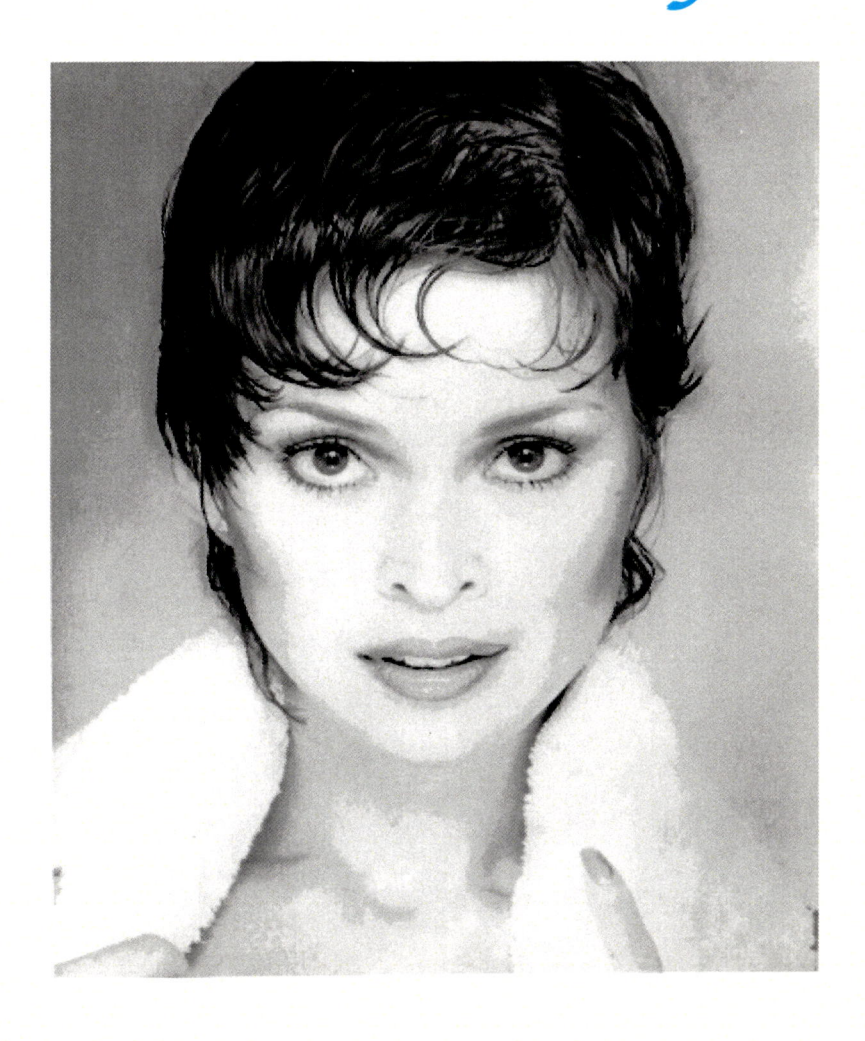

ANGEL IN MY POCKET

BY: JERRY SCHAFER

PUBLISHED BY BEGINNING II END PUBLISHING
800 N. RAINBOW #208
LAS VEGAS, NEVADA 89107

This autobiography is a tribute to Marianne Schafer, written by
her husband
Jerry Schafer

Cover design by Lee Brown
Editing By Aaron M. Angaran

ISBN
0-9706847-8-9
Copyright " 2002
All Rights Reserved
Printed in the United States Of America
August 2002

A Word From The Publisher

First of all, I would like to begin this forward by thanking Jerry Schafer for the opportunity to have had this up and close intimate look at his life, as the husband of Marianne Schafer. I feel not only privileged, but honored, in the event of having the chance for Beginning II End Publishing, Inc. to publish such powerful testimony and also the chance to meet your wife Marianne; not physically, but spiritually, through your words, stories and vivid pictures.

To all the readers who are fortunate enough to obtain a copy of this book, know that you are receiving these words, not by might but by fate. And once you read the compassionate, heartfelt words of Jerry Schafer, you will be able to use this book as a measuring device of what "true love" really is. I have used this story as one of my sculpturing components in my continuous journey to define my true, complete essence as a woman. I think this book should be read by anyone, who think they are truly ready to uphold the marriage vows in which many of us take for granted in this day and age. Their marriage is a true living testimony to the words; in sickness and health, for rich or for poor, till death do us part.

Then, when you dissect the two elements in what made such a beautiful marriage, you have a woman like Marianne Schafer. A woman who found the time to be a wife, raise children, cook, iron, grocery shop (with a list), do chores, assist her husband in business ventures, take care of finances, held a career as a model/actress and in all that still, found the time to be beautiful! Then, you take a husband like Jerry Schafer, a man who had wisdom enough to discern how awesome God was to bless him with a woman of this nature. He didn't take his wife for granted and out of his gratefulness, he showed her the utmost respect and demonstrated not only with words, but with action, true love and commitment. He chose Marriane in all aspects of his life; as a friend, a lover, a wife, a mother, a counselor, a spiritual advisor, his accountant and his business partner.

Thanks again, Jerry and Marianne, for giving us readers the recipe for true love and devotion. It has been an honor to preserve your marriage in the form of a book, which your testimony is truly worth being left, here on earth, until the end of time.

Yvonne Rainey
BEGINNING II END PUBLISHING INC.
CEO / Director

BEGUILING BEAUTY

*BEYOND HUMAN REASON OR REACH
SIMPLY STATED,
AN IMPOSSIBLE FEAT.
ONE WONDERS
AT THE INFINITESIMAL POWER OF
CREATING MARIANNE.
IT STANDS THEN
THAT ONCE KNOWN,
ONE COULD NEVER LET HER GO.
FOR SHE IS THE MIRACLE
THAT WE ALL CLING TO,
HOPE FOR AND BELIEVE IN,
SHE IS MARIANNE.
A TESTAMENT TO THE PROOF OF
A PERFECTLY FORMED UNIVERSE.
ONE THAT HAS THE POWER
TO CREATE PERFECTION ON EARTH.*

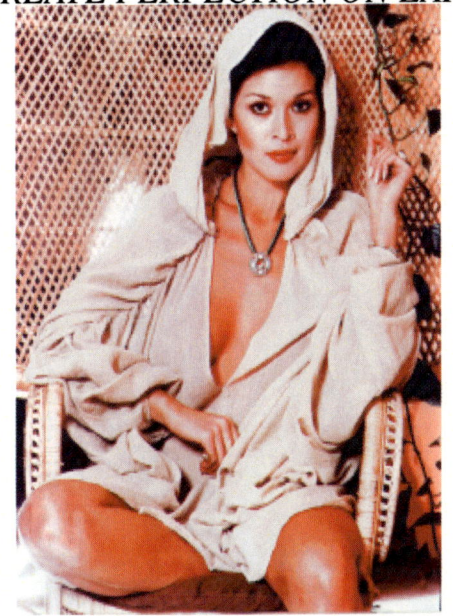

Jerry Schafer

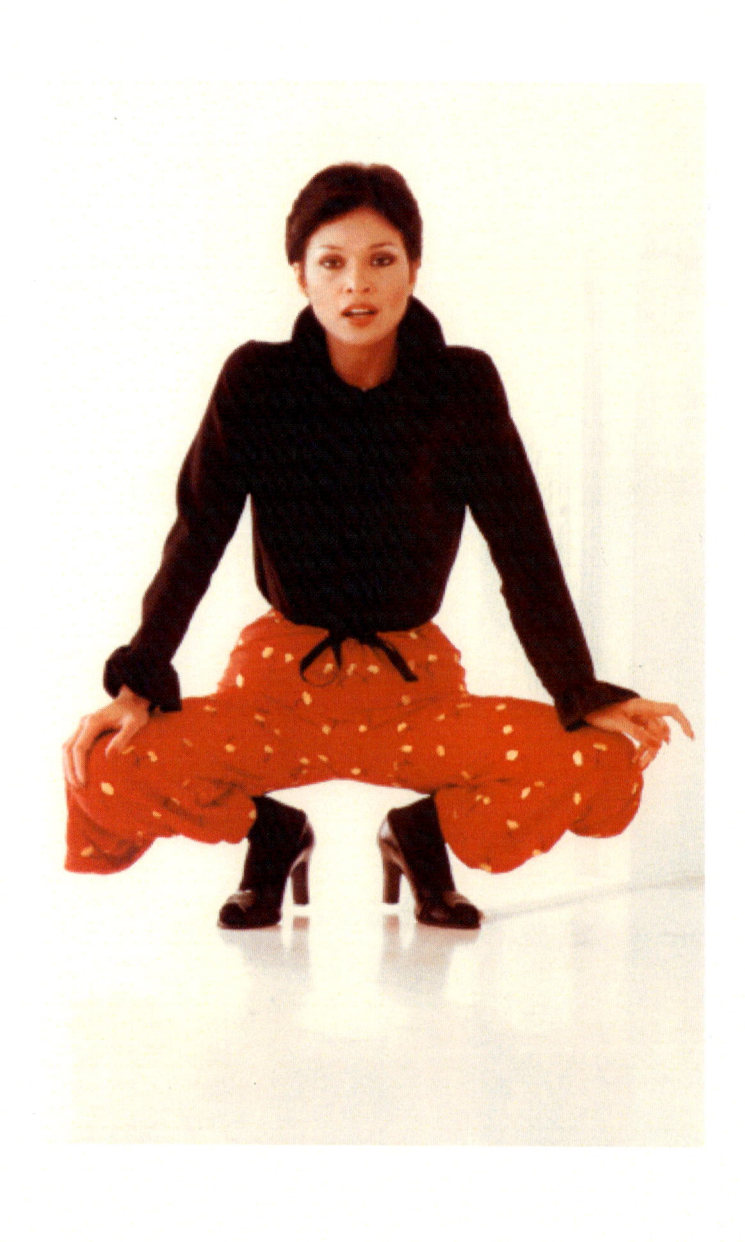

August 3, 2001

I received a phone call from Doctor Tafreshi at 6:30 P.M, advising me that I should go to the hospital and take Marianne home. His exact words were; "Mr. Schafer, the preliminary results of the biopsy on your wife's liver show that she has cancer of the liver!There's nothing more we can do. You may as well take her home!" I was in shock! "What does that mean, Doctor?" In a very cold manner the Doctor said, "I told you, there's nothing more we can do…so you should take her home!" Then, he hung up!

At approximately 7:30 P.M. I arrived at the Desert Springs Hospital with my friend Gordon Martines. Gordon went with me to help carry the flowers and other things that had accumulated in the hospital room.

It was almost 8:30 P.M. when we arrived at home. I helped Marianne get into bed. We were both in utter disbelief about the diagnosis. I held her and kissed her and told her, "I won't leave your side, honey, not even for a minute."

August 5, 2001

Today is Sunday. I have called Marianne's family and all five of my sons. I have advised every one of them as to what's going on.

Morgan and Mark offered to come to help at any time I needed them. They both said the same thing. "Just call, Dad and we'll be right there." My son Erik just returned from China. He was in Los Angeles. I spoke to him on Saturday and told him what was going on with Marianne. Erik began to cry.

I spoke with Doctor Pasha, a specialist, who was on Marianne's case in the hospital and told him what Doctor Tafreshi said to me. Doctor Pasha is going to the hospital tonight. He said that he will look at the results of the tests. He said he would call me tonight.

Meanwhile, at Marianne's request, I called a Catholic priest. He is coming to the house tonight to meet with Marianne, assuming he will give her communion.

As you can imagine, this is a nightmare for us. Through it all, Marianne is strong of will. She is very close to God. She always has been. I also know that Marianne loves me. Since the day we met, we have been inseparable.

I have nothing but love for her. That's not new. I've loved Marianne for twenty-four years. She is the light of my life, the star of my show, my best friend, my confidant, the only person I have ever completely trusted in my life. She is all things to me. If I lose her, life will have no meaning for me. I cannot imagine being without Marianne, even for a day, let alone for the rest of whatever time I have left on this earth.

Marianne has been a mother to my sons, a daily inspiration to me and, as I said, she is the light of my life.

Why God has decided to take her is inconceivable to me. Marianne could be the poster woman for any health magazine in existence. She works out daily. She doesn't drink or smoke. She takes carefully selected vitamins andminerals. She has a beautiful face and elegant body of an exotic beauty that she is. A most beautiful Island girl through and through. Her teeth sparkle. They are as white as the snow. In spite of it all, it seems her life is slipping away, like melting snow on the side of a mountain. Her courage is phenomenal, to say the least. She is strong of heart, strong of mind and quite set in her ways and beliefs. I have always tried to give Marianne anything that she wanted. Unfortunately, the most important thing I wanted for her I did not achieve. You see, her talents are boundless. I know how creative she really is. Marianne is a poet, a writer, a talented actress, a master chef and more. The list of her talents is endless.

During our marriage, Marianne has cooked me countless gourmet meals and served them to me like I was some kind of king. I thank God every day for letting me be married to a woman like Marianne. God has truly blessed me, to have had the moments we've shared together.

When I touch her hand, hold her or kiss her, I always feel as though I have to be really careful not to hurt her. I fear squeezing too hard or grabbing her too roughly, because that's what I really want to do. I love her so much, I could squeeze her so hard, it would hurt her.

She is a delicate flower and a raving beauty. As I have said, Marianne is my best friend, my lover and my wife. Marianne not only works hand in hand with me on every production that our company produces, she also washes my clothes, does the shopping, keeps the books, pays the bills, deals with all the telephone calls, designs the T shirts for our shows and does the jobs of at least five people. The list of her contributions to our marriage and to our business are endless. I have been able to ac complish a fantastic amount of productions, only because I have had the love, help, support, wisdom and talents of Marianne, behind every single thing I have done for the past twenty-four years.

To my children, she has been everything any child could ask for. She has always been there for them, no matter what. She has been more to them than just a mother. She has been a friend.

Marianne has an uncanny memory. She remembers everyone's birthday. I mean everyone we know. It's uncanny, to say the least. Her memory is boundless. I know it must sound self-serving, but Marianne is truly the most remarkable woman I have ever known. To our animals, she has been the finest mother that any domestic animal could ask for. Our dog, Banner, constantly looks through the window to see her inside the house and watch her moving about. When she is in the kitchen, he can't see that room, but he stares endlessly at the kitchen waiting to catch a glimpse of her. When he's inside the house, he watches her every move and follows her, wherever she goes. Our loving dog, Banner, died the following day after Marriane passed. I believe he felt her miraculous spirit move into a different realm of the earth and knew he must follow. Whereever she is, I know he is not far behind.

Like I said before and I'll say again, this cancer is a nightmare. I feel so helpless in this situation. I am seeking a way to try to save her life. I find myself looking for alternatives that Marianne will acquiesce to. Marianne told me that she does not want to take chemotherapy. She said, "You know, honey, I saw first hand the results of what it did to my mother and my father." Both of her parents died of cancer. Marianne told me the results of chemotherapy was devastating to her parents. Marianne hugged me close. "I just want to maintain the best possible quality with what's left of my life, honey. Please go along with me." My heart sank. Marianne knew there was no question that I would support any decision she made. I have always respected Marianne and her wishes.

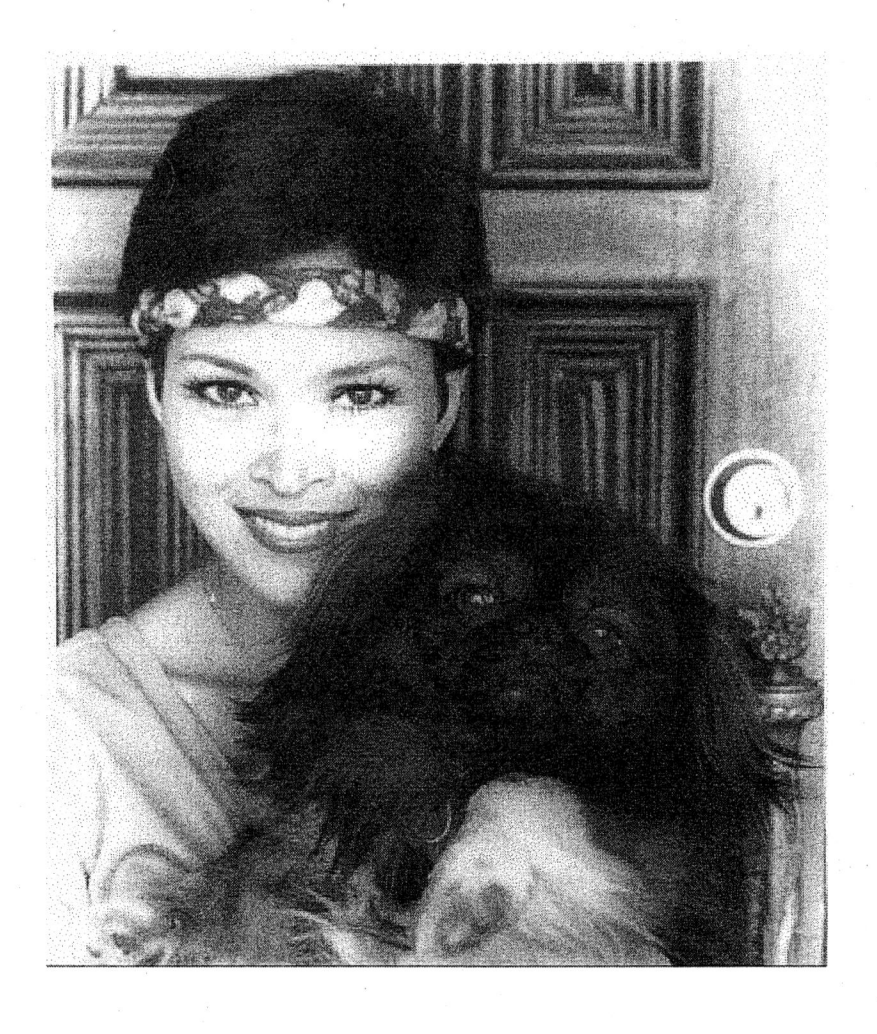

August 6, 2001

We know about a metaphysical method that a friend of ours feels can stop this horrible disease in its tracks. Marianne and I have been told that this method works. Our friend told us that he has seen it be successful with three people. Marianne smiled at me. She said, "It isn't chemotherapy, so lets give it a try!" The bottom line of this method, which I refer to as metaphysical, is 'Electronics in Medicine.' We have been told that electromagnetic and alternating magnetic energy of low power, properly tuned and/or applied, normalizes diseased tissue and can eradicate Marianne's cancer.

August 7, 2001

I have spoken with the people who have the machine that gives off the alternating magnetic current. I have requested their help and asked that it be used on my Marianne.

August 8, 2001

Marianne took the first test. The wheels are in motion to bring this metaphysical phenomenon to our house, as soon as the analysis is completed.

Today, Marianne is having pain. She took pain pills for the first time. She is so strong and so completely centered on what is happening to her that, as I said before, it makes me feel completely disarmed in every way. This continues to be a traumatic, heartbreaking period of time.

Through the night, I lay awake and watched her sleep. I wonder why God has elected to put her to this test. She is so beautiful when she sleeps, so tiny, so delicate and most of all, she is so good.

Every time one of my friends or acquaintances asks me about her, I begin to cry. I have begun to wonder if I'm feeling sorry for myself. I also wonder if I have any right to feel anything at all for myself in this situation. It is a ghastly feeling of helplessness. It brings into focus the lesson we all must learn. We are 100% powerless! That's what!

Oh God, please help my Marianne. Don't let her suffer. Wouldn't you know, that in the midst of this crisis, Marianne and I have a show in rehearsal. I cannot focus my attention on the show. With the expense looming on the horizon, Marianne and I need to generate whatever income we can. I must find a venue for this show, but, as I said, Marianne is the only thing on my mind.

August 10, 2001

Marianne is on the Machine! Wires are everywhere, connected to a large black belt that is fastened around her waist and chest area. Lots of lights keep flashing on a tiny box that is the control center of the machine. It looks like something out of a Twilight Zone program. God, I hope it really works!

I took Marianne to the cancer clinic today. The doctor prescribed medicine that has alleviated the pain. Last night, Marianne got a good nights sleep, without pain. The machine is still connected to her tiny body.

August 11, 2001

It's 9:45 A.M. Marianne is sleeping. I must go to rehearsal. Today, I will try to bring Jerry Aerola into the rehearsal hall, so that he can see the progress of the show. Marianne and I want to make an arrangement with him for publicity, no matter where we open.

Rene De Haven is doing a great job on the choreography. But, as usual with a live show, one of our best dancers is going to leave. We only have a few days left of rehearsal to teach a new, boy dancer the routines...that is, if we can find one that is good enough to do this intricate choreography. I will keep my cell phone in hand at all times. Marianne knows to call me, if she needs anything.

August 12, 2001

The Metaphysical Machine is still connected! Another friend suggest that we try hypnotherapy by an Israeli, named Ronnie Cohen. Ronnie was introduced to me by a fellow, named Hadar Orien. Hadar recommends Ronnie as being very good at his profession. He tells me that Ronnie has saved lives through his hypnotic techniques.

I hope that Marianne is receptive to this and that it can play a part together with the electronic machine in her complete recovery.

August 13, 2001

Well, it didn't work! Marianne did not take to the hypnotherapy at all. Ronnie didn't convince her that his technique would help. This morning, Marianne told me that she did not want to do hypnotherapy so, that's that! So much for that idea.

Please, God, let this Electronic Medicine work. Marianne is getting sicker. Thankfully, she sleeps off and on, but when she is awake, she is in pain and very uncomfortable. She is having so many trepidations about one thing or another.

"I'm so sorry honey," she keeps repeating, over and over again.

I feel like I am going to crumble, from the heartache this is causing. I love her so much and I am so helpless!

My son, Erik may come here today. He has been living and working in Taiwan. He is in the USA for a visit. So far, two phone calls have come to the house from a girl in Taiwan, who is worried about him. Erik is a real life Don Juan.

Last night, Erik called. He said that he would be here tomorrow or the next day. Marianne really loves Erik. She raised him through much of his adolescence. She has done many things for Erik, including buying him his first car. Marianne loves all the boys. She has never let any of them down, whenever they have had problems. I know how much she loves them all and I know they love her.

August 16, 2001

Greer Childers came here yesterday to help out and to be with Marianne. Greer brought us a "juicer". She showed me how to make healthy drinks for Marianne.

Greer is wonderful and I am so grateful to her for her compassion, her prayers and her juicer. She is coming back tomorrow to stay with Marianne, so I can go to rehearsal for an hour or so. I also have to shop for a few items.

August 17, 2001

Marianne had a bad night. I think we gave her too much carrot juice, because her mouth broke out with small sores from the acid. We will cut down the amount she drinks today.

Greer will be here at 11:45 this morning. I made another mistake yesterday, by giving Marianne a little milk. She has a lactose intolerance and it made her sick to her stomach.

I mopped the floors this morning and cleaned the kitchen. For the first time since I've been married to Marianne, I turned on the dishwasher (after Marianne told me how to do it). I sat in the chair, after I finished the housework and watched her sleep.

Rosey Grier called from Los Angeles to pray for Marianne. He has called every day since he found out about this insidious disease. Our friends Rosell Owens, Clancy Rail and Captain Snyder were here this morning.

They brought me some oatmeal and a turkey sandwich, which Marianne asked for. She asked me to order it for Greer. I know Greer won't eat it, but I ordered it anyway.

I don't think the machine is working. I'm not sure, mind you, but I know in my heart that God is the only chance we have. God has always been the only chance. To save my little Marianne, will take a miracle that only God can perform.

I am so tired now. I have stayed awake for eleven nights in a row. I'm afraid to stop watching her. I feel even more helpless, to help my Marianne. Every time I pray for help, I end up crying like a baby.

I'm keeping the house as clean as I can. I go into the bedroom every few minutes just to check and make sure Marianne is comfortable.

August 18, 2001

This morning, Marianne asked me to make her a bowl of mushroom soup. She ate it all. I am trying to believe that this progress is a result of the alternative electronic medicine. Whatever it is, now and always, as I have said, it will be up to God to grant us a miracle.

Marianne's friend, Sandra called from Utah. She offered to send us some kind of drink from Tahiti that may help Marianne. I asked her not to send it. Marianne is so sick and so tiny and so delicate, I'm afraid after the incident with the carrot juice, that the wrong thing in her body can do terrible damage to her. I explained this to Sandra. She said she would check into this and try to discover the ingredients. She said she would let me know what they are. It seems that many people have heard of ways to cure cancer. Unfortunately, the kind of cancer that Marianne has, is described by her doctor as the most insidious cancer of them all. They call it small, cell cancer. It is a horrifying killer.

My emotions are shot to hell. I'm so exhausted, that things seem unreal. God, I wish this were a bad dream!

I sat in the chair again last night and watched my Marianne sleep. She looks like an angel, as she lies there. How unfair it all is. Why such a beautiful, talented, wonderful woman like Marianne had to contact this insidious disease, is something that I will never understand.

August 19, 2001

Yesterday, was the best day so far. Marianne seemed to be in good spirits and didn't have too much pain or sickness to her stomach. Greer came over again and sat with Marianne. They talked for the longest time. When Greer left, Marianne seemed happier and more relaxed.

After putting in eighteen hours of going back and forth into the bedroom tending to Marianne, looking in on her in between bringing her something, pouring her water, giving her a pill, checking the electronic device etc., I am completely exhausted.

As long as Greer is here, I decided to relax for awhile. I sat on the couch in our dining room and turned on the TV. I have no idea what was on, but I sat there staring into the glowing, picture tube.

Suddenly, I heard a noise that sounded like someone was walking in our entry. I turned around and there stood Marianne, with a big smile on her face!

She began talking with an Irish brogue. I was dumbfounded. "What are you doing out of bed?" I asked. Again, using the Irish brogue, she said that she came out to water the plants. And she did! I just sat there in disbelief and watched her. Then, quietly, she went back to bed and fell asleep.

God, I pray that this machine is working. It seems as though it is. Her color is better and she seems stronger. Between giving her special drinks comprised of carrots and other vegetables (that I squeeze in the juicer that Greer brought) and with the machine and lots of love and attention, Marianne seems to be getting better. Tomorrow, I have to take her to the doctor at 10:30 A.M. I wonder what Doctor Allen will tell us. Even if the Doctor continues to say that this horrifying disease is killing Marianne, I won't believe it. I believe that God will perform a miracle. Between God, me and the prayers of friends, I pray that my Marianne is going to get well. When she does, I am going to take her to Hawaii and sit by the ocean with her and take pictures of her.

AUGUST 20, 2001

This morning, Marianne had two tablespoons of macaroni salad and a cup of tea. That was it! I am taking her to the Doctor at 10:30 this morning.

Today, we expect the report of how the electronic medicine is going. It seems as though it is working, at least on paper. Marianne is still in pain, but she told me it's not as bad as it was. She feels sick to her stomach most of the time.

Once in awhile, she gets a spark of energy. She will get out of bed, walk into the front room or the kitchen, doodle around for a few minutes and then, she goes back into the bedroom and falls asleep.

This is truly a nightmare, while being awake! Marianne is so brave and so controlled, in spite of what's going on. I am doing everything I can to keep her spirits up. At the same time, I think it also helps me to be strong, by trying to be strong for her.

God must be tired of me by now. I find myself asking for a miracle every few minutes, no matter what I'm doing. I can't help thinking that this must be what other people in this situation do. How could they do anything else?

When you love someone like I love Marianne, it rips your heart out every time you think about the inevitable.

After our visit to the cancer clinic today, it seems as though the doctors have given up. What the hell, they <u>have</u> given up! I am now convinced that medicine given to patients for cancer is just like paint by numbers. Whatever the situation calls for, there is a set pattern or group of tests that determine how the doctor treats the case. If the laboratory reports are too negative, like in Marianne's case, they simply tell you that it's a question of time. There is nothing more they can do! Then comes the question; "How much time does she have, doctor?"

The answer is part of the paint by numbers question and answers section. Regrettably, the doctor says, I can only guess. The fact of the matter is, it's up to God!

I can see that the doctors keep prescribing things or doing needless tests, even if they know it's a hopeless case. Back to square one. Money is the root of all evil!

In spite of this, Doctor Allen, at the Cancer Clinic, seems like a real square shooter. I will write what she tells me, when we return from our visit this morning.

12 Noon: We have returned from the visit with Dr. Allen. She told us that no further visits are necessary! She wants to make arrangements with a Hospice for them to send nurses to our house to help me keep Marianne comfortable. I told them no way. As far as I am concerned, Marianne is not about to die...not now!

Meanwhile, Robert Ahmanson, a friend of Marianne's, called. He wants to get the UCLA Medical Center involved for a second opinion. Robert made arrangements for the head doctor at UCLA to call today. He called and spoke with me and with Marianne.

Marianne and I discussed going to UCLA for a second opinion. It makes sense. What do we have to lose. We're not sure the machine is working...we're not sure of anything, except that Dr. Allen has given up.

The UCLA doctor will speak with Dr. Allen here in Las Vegas and will call us back in two days. If necessary, Bob said that he will send his jet to pick us up and take us to UCLA.

August 21, 2001

This morning, at 10:00 A.M. Zac Adelson brought a Rabbi to the house to pray for Marianne. What a lovely man he was. Young, spiritual and very smart. He also prayed with me and he put two mezuzahs on our house, at the front door and at our bedroom door.

Sam Fisher made special spaghetti for Marianne. I was thrilled to watch her eat. She actually ate more than at any time in the last eighteen days.

As promised, Bob called. He has arranged for Marianne to see doctor Lee Rosen at 12 noon on Thursday the 23rd, in Westwood, California. The appointment is at the Bowyer Oncology Center located in Westwood, California, near UCLA. Marianne cannot fly on a commercial jet, so Bob Ahmanson is sending his Citation to pick us up at 10:00 A.M. on Thursday morning. All I can say about this man, is that he is a very special person. Marianne adores him. The mention of his name always brings a smile to her face. I have known Bob for a little over twenty years. Bob told me I wouldn t have to rent a car. He said that when we arrive in Los Angeles, he will make arrangements to drive us to the doctor s office. After the visit, we will determine if we stay in Los Angeles or immediately, return to Las Vegas.

When we are in Los Angeles, I know that Marianne wants to see the ocean. Yesterday, she said, I really miss the ocean, honey! Why don t we drive down to the beach, after the doctor s visit?

We used to live in Malibu. It s no wonder that Marianne misses the ocean. I will arrange things so that we spend as much time as possible by the ocean, when we are in Los Angeles. In the back of my mind, I thought, my God, this could be the last time Marianne will see the **ocean.**

We talked about our cat. When we go to Los Angeles, our cat will be on its own for a couple of days, but we know that she can take care of herself. She sleeps 80% of the time, anyway. We decided to leave her enough food and water. After all, we only plan to be gone three days, at the most.

The report on the electronic medicine is in. According to the report, one of Marianne s cancers is gone, completely gone! I wonder if it s really true. The report also said that the other one is smaller, by one-third. We will connect the machine tonight and let her stay on it, until we have to leave on Thursday morning.

God, please grant the miracle I am praying for. Please cause these machines to have the power to make Marianne get well and give her back her life.

Greer was here tonight with her friend, Maria. They sat with Marianne, while Richard Lo Presto and I went to a local diner to get a salad. I told Marianne I would be gone for about 30 minutes. It was the first time I have left the house at night in eighteen days.

At the restaurant, I told Richard about Marianne s condition. I told him that I can t believe this is really happening. It s like a bad dream! Marianne is the only thing on my mind. I couldn t eat a bite of food. I ordered a salad to go and brought it home. Marianne was too tired to eat, but she said she would eat it tomorrow.

It is now 1:30 A.M. Marianne is sleeping but she is very restless. She is making strange little noises that scare the hell out of me.

As usual, I cannot sleep. Even while I write these notes, I keep going downstairs every few minutes and look into our bedroom to make sure she is OK.

I can t help thinking about this doctor in Westwood. What can he do? Is he for real? Is he seeing Marianne to placate Bob Ahmanson?

I remembered Dr. Allen s words: You don t have to return to our office anymore. There s nothing more we can do let us call the hospice and have them arrange to send someone to help you at home! My God, her words keep pounding in my head!

Can Doctor Allen be wrong? Was Doctor Tefreshi wrong? Was Doctor Pasha wrong? Is Doctor Liker going along with what he has been told to him by these Las Vegas doctors? How many opinions will it take to make me believe that God is going to take Marianne away from me and the world?

She has so much to offer. God knows that since 1992 we have put our combined talents into the development of the most prolific program ever to be produced about our nation. We also put every cent we saved into the *United States of America Series*, so we could make a contribution to our country and to the world, through educating people all over the globe about our great nation. That has been our dream. Marianne has worked tirelessly on this project. She wants to use some of the profits to help homeless people and disadvantaged children.

Our motives are so pure with this project. Oh, God, how could I ever do it without Marianne. Her talents are so important to this project. Her physical presence is also a major element in the production plan.

The other day, Marianne brought it up and we talked about it. You ve got to make the series, she said.

"If I'm not here in person, I'll be with you in spirit. You will hear me talking to you." She said, "I love you, Jerry. I have always loved you."

"I love you too, honey. God knows how much I love you." I kissed her and hugged her close to my chest. I closed my eyes and started to cry. I didn't want Marianne to know I was crying, so I pretended that I got something in my eye…she knew the truth though. I know it.

I told her that if I achieve the finance and if I can find the strength to do this without her, I would dedicate the series to her memory. I told Marianne that I will open the show with a full screen picture of her beautiful face over the American Flag. "The whole world will see my Marianne," I said. Marianne knows that by dedicating this series to her, it will put her name in history, until the end of time. She also knows that the series will be released around the world in 31 languages. God knows that without Marianne, I could never have put this monumental series together. She crossed the T's and dotted the I's and added her wonderful creative ideas to the project. As an example, Marianne created a new word that will be added to the dictionary, when she wrote: *"THE UNITED STATES OF AMERICA SERIES WILL BE THE HEIGHT OF "EDUTAINMENT."* Combining Education and Entertainment into a new word!

When it comes down to it, I imagine that everyone caught up in this kind of a situation prays to God that the doctors made a mistake. Or, maybe the laboratory made a mistake. Please God, let there be some mistake in this diagnosis. If there is no mistake, then chances are, I will spend the rest of my life alone. Without Marianne, there is nothing for me. I know I've said this earlier, but the thought keeps going through my mind.

Today, Bob Ahmanson called. He said that he was bringing his secretary, Fran on Thursday. I told Marianne that Fran was coming. Marianne smiled. "I'm glad," she said. "I really like her. She's a wonderful woman."

God, please don't take my Marianne!

Angel In My Pocket

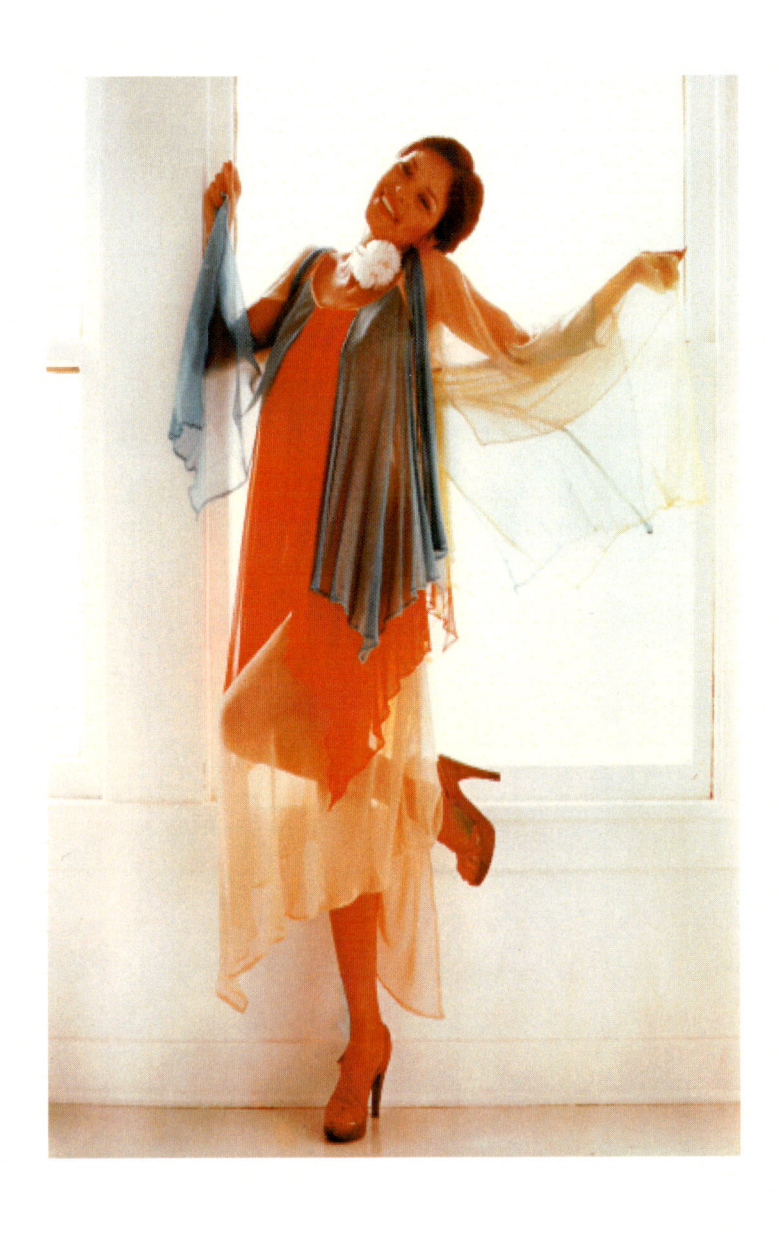

August 22, 2001

Marianne has had a bad morning. She is having pain. This sickness is getting to her. The terrible thought of what has been foretold, is becoming too much for her.

Sam Fisher is here to help me out. Greer said she is coming over this afternoon.

Bob called and asked if we needed a wheelchair for tomorrow. I asked him to speak to Marianne. She told him yes, she did need a wheelchair. Marianne asked me if we could spend the night in Los Angeles. I told her that Bob invited us to stay at his guest house and I had accepted the invitation. That really made Marianne happy.

Bob has a twenty-four hour registered nurse on duty for his wife, so the nurse will be moments away, if Marianne should need her.

After we finished talking about staying in L.A. overnight, Marianne smiled. She took my hand. "Don't forget, honey, we're going to the ocean, right?" "You bet we are," I said. "We're going to walk in the sand."

Sam Fisher came over. He had gone to the restaurant and brought us two club sandwiches with French fries. I fixed a tray for Marianne. She sat up and began eating French fries! Then, she ate a piece of the club sandwich. She even drank two cups of strawberry malt. I added ten drops of Noni, a drink from Tahiti that was sent here by Sandra, Marianne's girl friend, who lives in Utah. The stuff is supposed to have magical powers. God knows I'll try anything at this point.

August 23, 2001

We arrived at the UCLA annex at two in the afternoon. Marianne was in the wheelchair. I wheeled her into the waiting room and after a few short questions, we were ushered into the examination room. Marianne was sitting on the examination table. Bob Ahmanson was standing next to her. My friend, Moti came to be with us and he was also seated in the room. I was just behind Marianne. Fran, Bob's secretary, was also in the room.

After a few moments, Dr. Rosen walked in. Please, God, I prayed, let this man have the power to save my Marianne. Doctor Rosen was young and good looking. I wondered how such a young man could have the reputation he had as a maven, regarding this horrible disease.

Doctor Rosen told Marianne that he had examined the results of the biopsy taken in Las Vegas. He also said that he had two additional doctors check the results. He said he felt he could extend Marianne's life and possibly put the cancer into remission by using chemotherapy, combined with experimental medicine.

As you know, Marianne had already made it quite clear to me that she did not want to take chemotherapy, because of what it did to her parents. For some reason though, she looked at the doctor and said, "OK, Doc, lets give it a try!" I couldn't believe what I was hearing. The doctor ordered an ambulance and within fifteen minutes, Marianne was taken to the UCLA Medical Center.

August 30, 2001

Today, we returned from Los Angeles. Marianne received three rounds of chemotherapy, along with God knows how many tests, including, but not limited to, MRI's, CAT scans, PET scans, special shots, X rays and the list goes on…and on!

Bottom line, they saved her life! Dr. Rosen told me that without having the medicine they gave her, Marianne would not have lived past the end of the month.

Marianne had a very large room in the hospital. She was also given great care from an assortment of wonderful nurses and doctors. She was really a trooper, to say the least. She weathered the storm and never said no to any treatment suggested. At one point, she had six different chemicals dripping into her veins from needles placed in both of her arms. Talk about go with the flow. God, she was wonderful. I am so proud of her bravery and intelligence.

The second night in the hospital, I was hugging her and kissing her. Marianne began to whisper to me. "Honey, she said, I think I'm going to die tonight. I think this will be my last night on earth!"

Needless to say, I became a complete basket case, when she whispered those words into my ear. I called the priest and the doctor. The doctor assured me that Marianne would not die in the night. "Maybe," he said. "If a lightning bolt comes down something bad could happen but I doubt it.

I called the priest anyway. He gave Marianne the

last rights.

Thankfully, the doctor was right. I sat up all night and watched Marianne sleep. She woke up in the morning and everything seemed OK...or as OK as it could be, under the circumstances.

The next couple of days found Marianne being subjected to one test after the other, while bags of drugs were still dripping into her arms.

Once, I went for a walk, while she was sleeping. When I returned to the room, the bed was gone! I ran to the nurse's station. I was really scared. I asked the duty nurse where Marianne was. Oh, she said, she's down in X-Ray. She will be back in her room in about an hour. I took a deep breath and went to the pavilion. I sat on a bench. Being alone at a time like this is not easy. As I sat on the bench, taking in the California sun, mixed with smog, the world just seemed to stop. Something inside me said Marianne will beat this thing. I prayed to God and asked again, that he grant a miracle. I know that God loves Marianne.

I went back up to the ninth floor and into Marianne's room. There she was, sound asleep. She was exhausted from all the tests. I assumed my usual position on the couch and sat there watching her sleep.

The next day, the chemotherapy began. Marianne had three rounds (as they call it) of chemotherapy, over a period of three days. This was administered with some new, experimental drug. Thank God, Marianne did not get sick.

The doctors came into the room on the last day of

the chemotherapy and said I could take Marianne home. I called Bob and told him that Marianne would be released just before noon. He sent his secretary to the hospital. She drove us to Bob's house, where we spent the night. Bob arranged for a nurse to stay with Marianne all night. The next day, we took a private jet back to Las Vegas. We arrived home at about 12:30 in the afternoon on Friday, the last day of August.

September 1, 2001

Greer Childers arranged for a woman to help us out. This woman is named Maria and she is wonderful! She cleans, cooks and knows how to assist Marianne in every way. Taking care of Marianne is no easy chore. It takes lots of walking from the kitchen to the bedroom, lots of care in every way. Maria seems to be an expert in this regard. I found out that she has worked for five years with a woman who had cancer.

Maria told me that the woman she took care of, lived for 20 years, after the Doctors gave her just a few months to live. That's inspiring! That's the kind of stuff we want to hear. It gives us hope.

September 2, 2001

As Doctor Rosen predicted, Marianne is showing improvement in strength. This morning, she asked for a special drink that Clancy brought to the house. This drink is filled with supplements, that are just what Marianne needs. I made her the drink and served it to her. About ten minutes later, I turned around to find her walking down the hallway and into the kitchen with the empty glass! That's real progress, considering that Marianne has been flat on her back for almost a month now. She's still weak. I can barely hear her, when she speaks. No matter. I thank God throughout the day. I can see that she is improving.

Now, the battle begins. I made up my mind that I will find every kind of supplement known to fight cancer. I will add it to her drinks and food. I have already started by adding "Noni," that we got from Marianne's friend, Sandra. Like I said before, this stuff is supposed to be a magical, cancer fighter.

An acquaintance of mine said he knows of some stuff that he will get for Marianne. He sent me a fax with the information. This stuff looks like a real miracle. It's called MGN-3. It is supposed to kill cancer cells very quickly. I am praying that the combination of what the Doctors are doing, combined with Marianne's desire to win this battle and the supplements that I will find and give to her, will do the trick.

September 3, 2001

Last night was quite different. Marianne woke me at 3:00 A.M. and we went into the kitchen, where she ate a half of teaspoon of chocolate ice cream, a half teaspoon of vanilla ice cream and we went back to bed. After about ten minutes of conversation, she fell asleep. For the first time in many nights, so did I.

At approximately 5:15 A.M., I was startled to hear Marianne yell out. While I was sound asleep she got out of bed and went into the bathroom. She fell against the sink, knocking over several bottles of perfume and other stuff that was sitting on the sink. I rushed in, picked her up (thank God she didn t break anything) and carried her back to bed. I held Marianne s little face in my hands, For God s sake, honey, don t try to get out of bed without asking me to help you. I kissed her cheek. I didn t want to wake you. she said. Y ou haven t slept for so many nights.

I asked her what happened. She told me it was dark and she fell. That s that! Tonight, I will install nightlights in the bathroom, so that will never happen again. I also vowed to myself not to sleep at night, no matter what!

Today, Marianne s brother, Fred is arriving from Portland, Oregon. Marianne told me that she may ask Fred to help sort certain paperwork out. I may ask him to help or I may not, she said. It all depends on how I feel about it when I see him.

If she does ask for his help, I m sure Fred can handle whatever Marianne has in mind. I m also sure that Marianne has reservations about asking him to do anything, except visit.

September 5, 2001

Marianne is up and around! Just like that, she got out of bed this morning, got dressed, ate breakfast and began doing things around the house, just as if none of this had ever happened. It is really unbelievable. God is answering my prayers and the prayers of so many people, who have been praying for Marianne s recovery. I must admit, I m in total shock! It s really unbelievable. I know how deadly Marianne s cancer is. I also know that we have to go back to UCLA at the end of this month, for three more rounds of chemotherapy.

The fact of the matter is, if the quality of Marianne s life is good or as good as it seems to be right now and if she stays out of pain and can function normally, what more could we ask? Another 20 years would please me! I only hope and pray that the doctors will find a solution to getting rid of the cancer, once and for all. Like I said earlier, I am searching every day for some kind of solution, a thing, a process, a flower, a plant, electricity, some kind of drink something.

Tomorrow, a fellow is coming here with some kind of special water. I know it sounds strange, but according to one of my best friends, he has seen this water do miracles. That s what we need for Marianne. A full-blown state-of-the-art miracle.

Today, Fred helped me cut down part of a large tree. So far, Marianne has not asked Fred to do anything. Fred told me he is waiting for her to ask. If Marianne asks me to do something, I will be happy to do whatever she asks. But he said, If she doesn t ask me, I will just go home. If she wants, I ll come back again at another time . What more could Marianne ask of her brother. I am very fond of Fred Rhemrev.

September 6, 2001

I believe that Marianne is continuing to make progress. She seems stronger today. Fred will leave tomorrow, returning to Oregon. I continue to ask God to cure Marianne. We need a miracle that only God can provide.

September 7, 2001

Fred left today. I drove him to the airport. Marianne seems to be continuing to improve in strength. From time to time, I can see that she gets tired. I have a hard time convincing her to lie to down and rest. She is very compulsive, to say the least. It seems as though she feels compelled to do things. I hope she doesn t crash (for lack of better words), as a result of not taking it a little easier.

Marianne s brother John and his wife and son arrived at 9:30 tonight. They also live in Oregon. It was quite a surprise! Marianne was delighted to see them. They visited for a few hours and then went to their hotel. John said they will come back to our house tomorrow and visit with Marianne.

September 8-9-10-11

As I said, John and his wife arrived here on September 7th. They spent part of the 8th and 9th here at our house. John and his wife cooked a fabulous dinner. Their son, William, went to the casino to gamble, while John and his wife visited with Marianne and me. Marianne is feeling a little better. Her energy seems better too. Thankfully, she has learned to lie down when she feels tired. Thank God for that! Today, we went for a little ride to the jewelry store to pick up a few items that Marianne had cleaned. We also picked up my broken, but now mended, money clip.

After the jewelry store, Marianne browsed around a women s store for a while. She bought a few things. She seemed happy in the store and smiled a lot. Naturally, that pleased me to no end. I love her so much. Through all of this, I must admit, that I have become emotionally exhausted. These past weeks are starting to take their toll. The unbelievable trauma of it all is devastating; the heartbreaking news about my Marianne having cancer, the desperate hours, while she was in the hospital here in Las Vegas, the incompetent doctors here, giving us the wrong diagnosis at first. That trauma was followed by the days and nights at home, after the hospital. As long as I live, I will never forget what seemed like an eternity of nights of sitting watching her sleep, listening to her every breath, praying she wouldn t die.

I tried my best to care for her. I looked after her every need, while looking for a miracle from God or alternative ways to save her life. I brought the priest here from our local Catholic church. Through a friend, a local rabbi came to the house for the second time and prayed with Marianne. He visited for quite some time. Marianne really enjoyed his visit. After he left, Marianne told me that she thought the rabbi was really smart and cute too, she said. Under her pillow, were five or six crucifixes. At the head of the bed, is a photograph of a painting of the Virgin Mary. It was time to return to UCLA. Bob flew down and picked us up. This time, I checked into the Tiverton House, located across the street from the hospital. I wanted to be within walking distance, just in case.

We had a good flight to Los Angeles. Marianne seemed in pretty good spirits and was ready to take the treatments. We checked into the hospital. Again, Marianne was given a very large room. While the treatments were taking place, I sat on the couch. From time to time, when Marianne would sleep, I would walk in the hallway.

I was actually starting to have hallucinations from lack of sleep and worry. Those days and nights, combined with what we went through in Las Vegas, are finally starting to take their toll on me.

Every day we receive phone calls from well-wishers, friends who ask about Marianne and pay their respects by offering prayers. Each call is a reminder of the awful truth of it all. At the same time, I have learned to use these calls to encourage myself to remember that this is in the hands of God. In my opinion, Marianne has developed the right attitude to beat this horrible monster.

Along this path of rebuilding her strength and health, I must make up my mind to be careful what I say, as far as almost anything is concerned.

Marianne is very sensitive. She was sensitive before this happened, but now, her sensitivity has increased a thousand times. Even the wrong kind of look can cause some sort of outburst that makes her question one thing or the other. My love and devotion to her is stronger than ever. Today, I took Marianne to the eye doctor for her yearly exam. She was perfect. No changes in her prescription. She had a few of her sunglasses adjusted, before we left. Through all of this sickness, Marianne is more beautiful then ever. She is gaining back the weight she lost (approximately 24 pounds). She is eating very well and she is resting, whenever she feels tired. Her complexion is unbelievable. Her face actually glows!

I find myself thinking about our next doctor s visit here in Las Vegas and pray that her blood test will be as good or better than the last one. That visit will be followed by going back to the UCLA Medical Center on September 23rd., where Marianne will be in the hospital for three days for more chemotherapy. I will check into the Tiverton House again, but I plan to spend my days and most of the nights in Marianne s hospital room.

September 12, 2001

Today, Marianne started out rather slow. I didn't sleep last night. I stayed awake with an ear ache and wrote all night. I also tried to clean up my office area. Marianne seems disturbed today. I am certain it is about something I said. She seems depressed, slow in movement. As unbelievable as this may sound, at around 4 o clock this afternoon, I found Marianne hanging clothes on the line. I asked her to let me do it, but she refused, saying that she could do it just fine. Then, she calmly told me that she was not going to go back to UCLA. Why should I go back there, anyway, she said. I'm going to die. All they're doing is prolonging the inevitable!

I couldn't believe my ears. What are you talking about? I asked. That doesn't make any sense. You're doing so much better, honey!

No, I'm not, she said. It's just an illusion. Marianne continued the negative conversation. I'm tired of it all, she said. I just want to die!

All of a sudden, out of the blue, Marianne had changed her mind. I couldn't understand it. I think the medicine in her body is making her behave this way. Like I have written, Marianne changed her mind from her original decision not to take chemotherapy, to agreeing to try it. Now, suddenly, she wants to stop!

I know how close to God Marianne is. Although this decision is breaking my heart, Marianne knows I will support any decision she makes. Certainly, I know that we are all going to die. The moment we are born we begin to die. In a strange sort of way, it seems that if

Marianne carries out this threat, she will be committing suicide, just because she has gone this far. Everything we have done, all the chemotherapy Marianne has taken, will be for nothing. All of my efforts, as clumsy and uneducated as they may be, will have been in vain. All of Bob Ahmanson s efforts and help will have been for nothing.

My words to Marianne will go down as nothing more than dramatized, lip service! Oh, God, I feel that I m being selfish, but God knows that I don t want my Marianne to die.

I said, Marianne, honey, what about all the people who love and care about you! She replied by saying that I am the only one who really loves her. Jerry, she said. You are the only person on this earth who really loves me. I know that and I love you too. Please try to understand I just don t want to go on!

What about your brothers and your sister? I asked. They have their own families, she said.

I can t describe how this makes me feel. I know so many people who really love my Marianne. The more we talked about it, the more Marianne kept saying that she believed that I am the only one who really loved her.

I know she knows how much I do love her; I have proven that time and time again, over a period of twenty-four years. Marianne knows that she is the light of my life. I don t want to sound dramatic, but I could actually feel my heart breaking during this conversation. I m hoping that Marianne is talking this way, because of the medicine. Maybe the medicine is taking a terrible toll on her thinking. Whatever the case may be, however this turns out, I will support Marianne and I will be with her, no matter what!

September 14, 2001

Yesterday, started out badly. Marianne could hardly walk. As the day progressed, she seemed to get a little stronger. By the end of the day, she was stronger, yet. As usual, she began to do chores around the house. I tried to stop her, but as usual, my dialogue fell on deaf ears. She continued to work in the kitchen and other places in the house. When she started to vacuum, I insisted that she stop. Thankfully, she did. I guess this means there will be ups and downs throughout the time we fight this disease. The up s and down s may continue, until Marianne beats it. I still believe that she will beat it. I pray to God throughout the day, to grant the miracle I have been asking for, from the beginning of this ordeal. Through it all, I believe that Marianne will survive this dastardly thing and become a national spokesperson in the fight against cancer. At least that s what I m praying for.

Yesterday, I received a letter from STOP DUI, a non-profit organization designed and dedicated to stopping the violent crime of driving under the influence and assisting the innocent victims of this crime. This is one of Marianne s pet peeves. A few years ago, we made a documentary on this subject and Marianne was the star and narrator of the show. It was a tremendous success and hopefully, saved lives. As a matter of fact, Marianne won the New York Television Festival for Best Narrator and Best Performance in a documentary with this show. Now, they are requesting that we make another, more comprehensive documentary on the same subject, to be submitted to police agencies and schools around the nation.

Marianne wants to be involved in this new project, by once again, being the spokesperson and narrator for it. No one could do a better job then Marianne. Hopefully, we will find the finance necessary to do this documentary and hopefully, the diversion of working may help to heal my Marianne.

    I have to take Marianne to the cancer clinic here in Las Vegas for her weekly check up and blood test. The last test was 5.7. They said it was very good. We hope this one is good, too.

September 15, 2001

I had to get a wheelchair for Marianne at the clinic. It was just too far for her to walk. She took the blood test and we waited for the results. It was awful! 0.7.

Dr. Allen s nurse gave us the bad results, but told us that was expected. Marianne s immune system is all but gone. The nurse said they will give Marianne five continuous days of shots. They said the shots will bring her immune system back, but will cause her to have pain in her bones and possible other pain.

My God, this is a nightmare for Marianne, but through it all, she continues to smile. Her bravery is unreal. This horror seems to be never-ending. One frightening dimension after the other. Marianne took two shots. One of them hurt her. It burned real bad, as it was injected into her. Tomorrow, she must have another, then the day after that another, followed by another!

I called Bob Ahmanson from the clinic and told him what was going on. As we were speaking, Marianne was finished with the shots. I handed her the phone, so she could speak with Bob. I knew that would divert her a little and take her mind off the pain she just suffered. I was right. The talk with Bob seemed to lift her spirits.

I helped Marianne into the our car. As we drove she started talking about getting more shots tomorrow morning. Then, she changed the subject and said, Lets go to the market. I want to do a little shopping!

As usual, Marianne was unpredictable. God, I love her.

We drove to Albertson s market. Marianne drives

an electric cart to do her shopping. This is the second time she has used this device. She s cute as hell, as she drives it all over the market. We also had to fill a prescription. The market has a drug store, so we killed two birds with one stone. Marianne bought some fried chicken. We ate it when we got home. Marianne continues to amaze me in as much as her bravery is concerned. She is one wonderful lady. God, why is this happening? Please, make it go away from my Marianne!

The following day, we arrived at the clinic about 9:30 A.M. Marianne went directly into the chemotherapy area where the nurse instructed her to sit in one of the large chairs. After about a fifteen minute wait, a nurse arrived carrying the injection she was about to administer to Marianne. She told Marianne that this shot was mean and that it was going to burn, as she injected her with the medicine.

I watched as the nurse took the needle and inserted it into Marianne s arm. The injection took about three minutes, as the medicine had to be injected slowly, because of its effect (pain), as it is being administered. Marianne just sat there and didn t move. I saw her grit her teeth, as the needle went in. Once in awhile, during the injection, she would grimace. I felt so helpless, watching my Marianne be subjected to this.

I spoke with one of the nurses, who told me that this was all part of the procedure, when chemotherapy is involved. The nurse said that the chemotherapy causes the immune system to break down, but, she said, These injections will restore Marianne s immune system! The nurse said she doubted that Marianne would have to con tinue with these shots, after this series of five injections. Remarkably, when we got home, Marianne seemed OK. She started doing things around the house. As for me, I couldn't get it out of my mind. I went into the back yard, pretending to clean things up, but what I really did was cry. I feel so absolutely helpless in this situation. It's driving me crazy. Why is this happening to my Marianne? A cold chill came over me. For the first time, I felt like this was going to be a losing proposition. My Marianne is going to die!

September 15, 2001

It's Saturday morning. I will take Marianne to the cancer clinic for her shots. The clinic wasn't too crowded this morning. Again, I stood there watching Marianne take this painful shot.

After we got home, Marianne didn't feel too well. No wonder! Who would? Marianne rested in the afternoon, but I knew that she was very upset with the whole thing. I told her how much I loved her. I kissed her cheeks and her eyes and ears and whispered to her, telling her how proud I am of being her husband. Every word I say to her is the God's truth. I know this is a living nightmare for Marianne. I wish I could take her pain away. As I go through this with her, it is nothing short of a living nightmare for me, too. I find myself questioning God. Why Marianne? Why this wonderful, talented beautifulgirl...why? I still didn't sleep all night. Marianne and I talked in bed until about 1:30 A.M., when Marianne asked me to fix her some eggs. I love to do anything for her. I always have. I went into the kitchen and scrambled up the eggs. As I was doing that, Marianne appeared and took a few other things and put them on her plate. After she ate, we went back to bed and Marianne fell asleep. But I couldn t sleep. My mind kept racing with thoughts of what I could do to save Marianne. Along with those thoughts were thoughts of the reality of what is going on. It is now 3:15 A.M. I sit here writing this, knowing that at 9:00 A.M. this morning, Sunday, September 16, 2001, I will take Marianne back to the cancer clinic for another one of those painful shots.

In six days, we travel back to Los Angeles. I talked to Bob and gave him our schedule. He said he will pick us up in his jet on Saturday the 22nd. Even though Marianne had changed her mind about going back to UCLA for some reason, she was going along with the schedule to return! Our discussion turned to our cat. We only have a few more days to decide what to do with Baby, our cat. We don t want to leave her alone for five days. Marianne will be in the hospital from the 23rd through the 25th. We will return to Las Vegas on the 26th or maybe the 27th..

I will continue writing this, after the shot this morning:

September 16, 2001

Marianne took the shot. This time, I actually felt her pain, as the nurse injected the hot fluid into her body. I went weak in the knees and got sick to my stomach.

After the shot, Marianne decided that she wanted to exchange a bracelet I had given her. She said that she wanted something else. So, we drove to the store. I could tell that Marianne was very weak. Thankfully, she agreed to use the wheel chair. It was a good thing, too, because she took her sweet time.

After approximately an hour, Marianne found what she was looking for, a beautiful bracelet and necklace. They look terrific on her. The truth is, everything looks terrific on her!

As the day passed Marianne had her ups and downs again. Feeling lousy for part of the time and feeling OK for the other part. A few friends called her and she talked on the phone with them. I always hope these phone calls give her added confidence and hope.

September 17, 2001

Our appointment at the Cancer Clinic is for 11:30 A.M. today. Another painful shot. When we return, I will continue this summary.

This time, Marianne smiled at me, all the while the nurse was injecting her. I couldn t believe my eyes. She just sat there and smiled! As I have told you, Marianne is really quite unbelievable, in every way. She told me it didn t hurt too badly today. I put my arms around her. As I hugged her and kissed her, I had a huge lump in my throat. I know that tomorrow we must go back to the Cancer Clinic at 2:30 P.M. for a blood test. This will tell if Marianne s immune system is functioning properly. If it is, the shot may not be needed. God I pray that is the case.

We have four days left before we venture back to Los Angeles. As I have said, on the night of the 22nd, we plan to stay in Bob s guest house. Bob told me that he has planned some fun stuff for the day. His help and support continue to be major factors in Marianne s mental attitude. I am very grateful to him.

Marianne didn t feel too well after having the shot. She had a rather slow morning both mentally and physically but in the afternoon she seemed to perk up a bit and went through the rest of the day quite well.

It is now 10 A.M. on the 18th and Marianne is still sleeping. She got up several times during the night. Hopefully she will sleep through much of the morning. I know that rest is good for her. I believe it helps to revitalize her system.

This overview will continue.

October 1, 2001

We have now returned from UCLA for the second time. Marianne took three days of chemotherapy. The doctor told me that this time the treatment was significantly stronger than the last time we were at the hospital. The doctor has increased the dosage because he said, Marianne is able to tolerate a larger dose now. Marianne is really a great patient. She went through the three days with a smile on her face. Crazy as it sounds, as I sat there each day and watched the nurses shoot her with needles, inject her with medicines that caused her lots of pain and suffering, Marianne seemed to sail right through it. But, not me. Watching this, has began to have a very bad effect on me. I am at my wits end, now. It s happening to my Marianne, but in the strangest sort of way, it s happening to me too.

As you can tell from the lapse of information between September 17th and October 1st, I was unable to write anything. The effect of this is unnerving, to say the least. Every day I write a letter to God, asking for mercy for my Marianne. After the hospital in Los Angeles, we returned to Las Vegas, via Bob s private jet. As usual, he was wonderful. He loves Marianne and does what he can to support her through this awful crisis.

Meanwhile, the trips to the Cancer Clinic here in Las Vegas continue. They still have to give her the horrifying shots, that are designed to repair her immune system. Now it has become a ritual. Marianne smiles at me, as they inject her. I crumble inside while I watch, but I won t let her know it. All I do know, is that I will not leave her for a moment. My attention to her every need has caused me to lose my focus in my business dealings, but frankly, I don t give a damn.

Today is our 23rd Anniversary! Like most people in this world, we ve had good times and bad times. We ve been very lucky to be in love like we are. Through the good and the bad, we have always been deeply in love with each other and that fact made everything else seem unimportant. We are really soulmates. Marianne has taken care of me for twenty-three years and I have tried my best to reciprocate. She is the apple of my eye and the love of my life and she always will be. In between thinking that Marianne will die, I still want to believe that Marianne will beat this cancer. I do believe that she can receive the miracle that I have been praying for. Please, Dear God, eradicate this disease from her body.

Today, at 2:00 P.M. we go to the Cancer Clinic for another shot. We expect to hear from doctor Rosen tomorrow, regarding a new, experimental medicine called Gleevac. If this medicine can be given to Marianne, it may be the answer to all our prayers. We will know tomorrow, after the doctor receives the reports from the laboratory, to discover if Marianne can tolerate this new medicine. He is making sure it will not interfere with her present treatment.

October 9, 2001

The past days have been filled with going to the Cancer Clinic. Some days, they give her two shots and other days, they draw her blood, on top of the shot. She is really taking this very well, in spite of the pain of it all. Marianne continues to be my hero. She is the bravest person I have ever known. God bless her for being so strong of mind and so close to you.

We must return to UCLA hospital on the 24th of this month. Marianne will have three more rounds of chemotherapy, together with additional tests, to see how well her liver is responding to the treatment. After this hospital stay, Doctor Rosen says he will try the experimental Gleevac on Marianne. This may be the magic pill that will kill the cancer in her body.

My daily prayers continue, asking God to grant Marianne the miracle of being cured, once and for all. I pray this medicine will be the answer. On top of my verbal prayers, my letters to God continue on a daily basis. Marianne s sister, Grace, visited us for two days. It was nice to see her. In answer to my calls, both of her brothers and her sister have come from Oregon to visit with Marianne.

November 28, 2001

Marianne has to go to the Cancer Clinic here in Las Vegas eight days per month. On top of that, we spend one week per month in the hospital in Los Angeles, where the chemotherapy continues, along with additional tests.

I am happy to say that Marianne is looking better and better every day. She is beginning to work out a little. As I said before, she is so brave and so strong through all of this, that it amazes me to no end.

The trips to Los Angeles, hospital, doctors, Cancer Clinic, etc., are costing us everything we have. I must get a show booked and fast. Marianne asked me not to go to the hospital in Los Angeles for the next round of Chemotherapy. Stay here, honey. You ve got to produce a show. We need the money!

At first, I said no, that I wouldn t let her go alone, but Marianne insisted. I ll be fine, she said. Bob and Fran will come every day and so will Beth I ll just take the chemo and use this visit to rest as much as possible. That s what she said!

I didn t want to argue with her and the fact of the matter is, she s right. We do need the money. We talked it over throughout the rest of the day and finally, decided that we must do our show. That means that I have to stay in Las Vegas and work, while my Marianne goes to UCLA without me.

Bob Ahmanson has helped out again. He brought the private jet here and flew Marianne to L.A. Then he took her to the hospital and got her checked in.

Don t worry, he told me. W e ll look after her just like she s my own daughter. You know that, Jerry. She will be just fine!

Bob said that he will fly Marianne home after the treatments, at the end of this week. All during the week, I was a total basket case. I called the hospital no less than ten times a day. I remained in Las Vegas, working on the show, getting it ready to open, but my mind was only on my Marianne. As it turned out, this hospital visit was devastating. They hurt Marianne badly. Too many needles in her little arms. Her veins have collapsed. They cannot stick needles into them anymore.

Dr. Rosen called me. He said that during Marianne s next visit to the hospital, they are going to operate on Marianne and install a Hickman Device into her body. The doctor tells me that will allow them to administer drugs, without putting any more needles into her arms.

December 26, 2001

Christmas came and went and we didn t even know it. Every year since I ve been with Marianne, she has sent Christmas cards to people all over the world. She never forgets anyone. But this year was different. Marianne was too sick to do anything and I was too busy taking care of her, to care about anything else. I haven t writ ten for some time now. I've been watching this horrible disease take its toll. One day Marianne feels OK. Thankfully, she has no pain. Then suddenly, the next day the pain is awful. The pain is in her back and her neck. She complains of pain in her head. I don't know what it is, but I know something is different and definitely wrong!

During the time I have been keeping this journal on my Marianne, I have tried to document what she has had to endure. I have watched her suffer the indignities, pain and suffering that goes hand-in-hand with small cell cancer, being in hospitals, etc. I have lived every moment with her, hardly sleeping at all, because I would rather just look at her all night, in case God decides to take her from me. I can't get enough of her, even if it means that I just look at her beautiful face. I never stop telling her how much I adore her. The fact of the matter is, I am, as I have been from the beginning of this nightmare, completely helpless. Each day, I find myself becoming more unsettled in my head and in my heart. My insides have a strange empty feeling. It is becoming more painful each day. It is also becoming obvious that my Marianne is dying a slow death.

For the past three days, I have tried to reach Doctor Rosen, but he is out of town. His answering service connects me to a doctor, who does not know Marianne. I am not happy with that arrangement. Marianne became so sick, that I finally did speak to this doctor and told her of Marianne's symptoms. She recommended that I take Marianne to a hospital here in Las Vegas. That scenario is unacceptable to me, as I am convinced that the Las Vegas medical community leaves something to be desired.

December 28, 2001

At 1:15 A.M. this morning, Marianne came into the bedroom and sat next to me. Honey, she said, I don't feel right at all. She told me that she had a terrible pain in her head.

I laid her down next to me and held her tight. Just rest, honey. Let me hold you. Try to relax. I kissed her cheek and patted her head, trying to calm her down. I love you, Marianne.

After a few moments, she smiled at me and kissed me. I was starting to believe that whatever was bothering her, would go away. Marianne was beginning to relax. She was holding my hand, when suddenly, she had a horrifying seizure! She began to jerk and twist. Her face twisted to one side and she passed out.

I called Doctor Rosen in Los Angeles. Thank God, he came to the phone immediately. He told me to take Marianne to the closest emergency hospital and have them give her a brain scan. I called my son, Aaron and woke him, asking for his help. Aaron arrived at our house within ten minutes. Aaron is a surgical technologist and knows a lot of people in the hospital.

We got Marianne to the emergency room within five minutes after leaving the house. Aaron had called ahead. As I pulled up to the Emergency Area, they were waiting for us with a wheelchair. As they were wheeling Marianne inside, she began to throw up. Her head went forward and I grabbed her, to keep her from falling out of the chair. Her face was as white as a ghost. The immediate diagnosis was that she had suffered a stroke. I called

Doctor Rosen and told him what they said. Doctor Rosen spoke with the doctor, at Desert Springs Hospital. After his conversation with the doctor he called me on my cell phone. He said, Jerry, I want you to get Marianne back to UCLA as fast as possible. Call Air Ambulance. I ll make arrangements at UCLA for your arrival!

It was about 3:30 a.m. when I finished making the arrangements for the air ambulance and two ground ambulances. On the way to Los Angeles, Marianne was unconscious. The nurse in the Air Ambulance kept her on oxygen all the way. During the flight, the nurse monitored Marianne with some kind of machine. As a matter of fact, that nurse never stopped writing and doing things to Marianne during the entire trip. The flight took approximately forty minutes. We arrived in Los Angeles at the UCLA Medical Center at approximately 5:30 A.M. on Sunday, December 29th. Marianne was admitted through the Emergency Area, where a team of five neurologists examined her. Then, she was taken to a room on the 4th floor. The Neurology Section of the hospital.

The next morning, on December 30th, at approximately 10 A.M., doctor had just finished examining Marianne. He looked at me and smiled. Things seem to be coming along just fine, he said, I ll be back in about twenty minutes. The doctor left the room. I noticed that Marianne had something on her tooth. I opened her mouth and with a damp wash cloth, I took it off. There, I said, You re beautiful again! I turned to the sink to wash my hands, when suddenly, Marianne sat straight up in the bed and let out the loudest, most horrifying scream, I had ever heard in my life. She was having her second and most devastating seizure. It rendered her unconscious for quite a long time. I was alone with her in the room, when it happened. She began to shake and tremble in an uncontrollable manner. I ran into the hallway and yelled for help. The nurses and doctors came running. They surrounded the bed, giving Marianne oxygen and stuck her with countless needles.

I had to sit down. I was completely exhausted, from being awake all night, being on the Air Ambulance, in two ground ambulances and in the hospital, where I stayed awake in the room, standing next to my Marianne, all night.

A doctor walked over to me and put his hand on my shoulder. Let me tell you something, Mr. Schafer, he said. These seizures are more frightening than they are dangerous. He assured me that they had given Marianne some medicine that should prevent further seizures. He did say there were no guarantees, though.

I continued staying awake, watching the drama unfold. Marianne couldn t speak. She was delirious the rest of the night. Nurses were in and out of the room every fifteen minutes or so, watching her closely.

The next morning, Marianne was examined by one doctor after the other. Doctor Rosen assured me that she was in good hands and by the following day, they would transfer Marianne to the 10th floor of the hospital, where they would proceed with her chemotherapy. Unfortunately, that didn t happen. Through a series of tests, including a spinal tap, the neurologist discovered that Marianne s cancer had moved from her liver to the fluid around her brain. That s what caused her to have the seizure.

Now, for the first time, I understood why Marianne had been complaining about having pain in her head, and neck. The small cell cancer had moved into her head, where it was preparing to take Marianne s life, in a most insidious way. The doctors told me that they would have to inject chemotherapy directly into Marianne s brain! I went weak in the knees. My God, I said. How can you do that? The doctor explained that they would have to perform an operation on Marianne s head. My first reaction was, no. I told them no. No operation on her brain. The doctor told me that this operation did not go into the skull. We don t have to operate on her brain, he said. We will simply make a small port on her head. He told me they do this procedure daily and he said it wasn t a big deal. It should only take about 30 minutes in surgery. After hearing all of the medical reasons why this was necessary, I finally relented.

After I agreed, the doctor told me that through the port, they can inject the chemotherapy directly into her head and it won t hurt her. There should be very little discomfort, he said.

I went with Marianne to the Holding Area just outside of the operating room. I held her hand and kissed her. I told her she was going to be OK and that I was going to stay right there, until she came out of surgery. That s exactly what I did. I stood outside the surgery for four hours! Not thirty minutes like I was told. Four hours! That s howlong it took! When they wheeled her out of the operating room, I could see a trail of blood dripping out of the bandage on her head. As I said, before the surgery, they gave Marianne a spinal tap. After the surgery, they injected chemotherapy directly into spine, as well as directly into her head. Needless to say, Marianne became very, very ill. She began to vomit uncontrollably. I have never seen anyone so sick and in such pain. I couldn t stand to watch any longer. I went outside the hospital. It was pouring rain. I walked and cried, for what seemed like hours. Actually, it was about forty minutes, before I could contain myself. I was crying, because I realized that I was watching my beautiful Marianne, as she continued toward the road to her death.

What could God be thinking about? Cancer in her liver was bad enough. That in itself, is a death sentence. But no, it seems that wasn t bad enough. Now, the cancer has traveled into the fluid around her brain and down into her spine. I thought, why, God? What are you doing to my Marianne?

The following morning, I walked out of the hospital like a zombie. I was completely exhausted, mentally and physically. As I was walking in the courtyard in front of the hospital, a man smiled at me. In a loud voice, he said, Happy New Year! My God, I didn t even realize that New Year s Eve had come and gone. I didn t care, either. I still don t. All I care about, is my beautiful Marianne. Bob Ahmanson came to the hospital and asked me if I intended to write a story about Marianne s life. It s already in the works, I said. I will call it, ANGEL IN MY POCKET.

I have always carried a photograph of Marianne in my pocket and she has always looked like an angel to me. She really is an angel, in so many ways. She is the most thoughtful person I have ever known. She never forgets anyone s birthday. In fact, Marianne never forgets any thing! Even the most casual acquaintance will be remembered by a card from Marianne. Bob is thinking that if something happens to Marianne it would be nice to have documentation about her life. Let s face it, something happens to all of us in our cycle of life. Remembering Marianne in writing is something that I would do anyway. People who know me, know that s a given.

I know it sounds crazy, after all I have told you so far; my Marianne, this insidious cancer in her body, the way I am seeing it kill her, etc., yet, in spite of it all, deep down inside, I keep praying that a miracle is on the way. Maybe it s Jerry s folly, but I refuse to believe anything, other than the fact that Marianne is going to get well. She will fool lots of people. At least that s my deepest hope inside my heart and my constant prayer to God.

I am writing this book, because I love Marianne beyond words. I want to leave a testament about her life as my gift to whoever reads it. In many ways, Marianne has led a wonderful and most, fantastic life. Marianne lived on three continents. Marianne Vermeer Rhemrev was born in Djkarta, Indonesia. When she was four years old, her family emmigrated to Holland. To this day, Marianne still carries a Dutch passport. Every time we went to a foreign country I d have to get a visa but not Marianne. Her Dutch passport let her travel the world without a visa. She told me once that she would never give up her Dutch passport. No wonder. If I had one, neither would I. Her, father William, was the light of her life. Her mother was her inspiration.

In spite of the fact that she couldn t speak one word

of English when she arrived in America within one year at her elementary school, Marianne became number one in her class. More about her life later.

January 16, 2002

We just returned from the Cancer Clinic in Las Vegas. Dr. Allen gave Marianne chemotherapy directly into her brain. After the injection, they removed the clamps from her operation. Doctor Allen called me aside. She took me into a small room.

I m sorry, she said, But Marianne is not going to live much longer! She went on to tell me that there wasn t any cure for the type of cancer that was in the fluid around her brain and in her spinal column. Dr. Allen suggested that I should make arrangements with the Hospice. How long will she live, I asked. I can t tell you for sure, the doctor said . It could be two weeks or maybe even a month. It felt like my heart stopped beating. I have been believing that Marianne was going to get well. Remember the miracle I ve been praying for? I began to cry. Dr. Allen put her arms around me. I m sorry, she said. Marianne is really an exceptional person. I m very sorry. She continued holding me and I continued crying like a baby.

Finally, I pulled myself together and went into the hallway, where Marianne was waiting in a wheelchair. She smiled at me and I kissed her on the head. Come on, I said. Lets go.

As I was wheeling her out of the clinic, I remem

bered when that other doctor told me that Marianne wouldn t live past the month of August. That was almost six months ago. In spite of it all, I still wouldn t accept the inevitable. Maybe Marianne will still fool them. Again, I thought, *God, why are you doing this to my Marianne?* I can t understand it. Why does this wonderful girl have to suffer like this?

As I put Marianne into our car, she looked at me and smiled. At that moment, I knew Dr. Allen had told her what the expectations were. I knew that Marianne had also accepted it.

We drove to a drug store with Marianne s new prescription. As I drove Marianne told me that she was ready to die. It s really OK, she said. I m proud that God wants me at this young age. I m worried about you, though, honey, she said. I had to pull the car over to the curb. I was so upset and frightened. Once again, I began to cry. I held Marianne in my arms and we sat there, cheek to cheek, for at least ten minutes. We didn t speak. We were both caught up in our thoughts. Finally, I was able to drive home.

I knew that Charlene was coming to the house to visit Marianne. I decided to take the prescription to the pharmacy, after I got Marianne home. She had enough excitement for the day. Charlene was waiting, when we arrived home. She looked after Marianne, while I went to the drug store to pick up the prescription.

Charlene is like an angel to both Marianne and to me. She has helped me look after Marianne this week, cooked for Marianne, even bought our dog a treat or two. This girl is remarkable and far beyond a friend. No rela tive could be this wonderful or thoughtful or giving. God has blessed us with her presence.

I just spoke to another wonderful friend, named Bonnie Sax. Bonnie is very spiritual and has prayer groups all over the country, praying for Marianne. She and her husband, Shelty, are coming to visit Marianne around 4 this afternoon. I am beside myself, trying to understand it all. Why? Why? For God s sake, Why?

January 20, 2001

Marianne had a very bad day yesterday. January 19th was the worst day so far. She was in terrible pain most of the day. I gave her the new pills, but they just don t seem to work. Marianne s friend, Sandra Wolfson, from Utah, flew in to see her. Sandra has been a friend of Marianne s for twenty years. They held hands and talked for quite a while.

My son, Aaron and his wife and daughter, came over. Melanie visited with Marianne. Then, Charlene & her husband came by. Mike Tessaro, Charlene s husband, came over to cut Marianne s wig. Naturally, it was Marianne s request and Mike wanted to accommodate her. At first, Marianne insisted that she would sit up and have Mike cut the wig while it was on her head. What a mistake! God, love her. She tried. She put on the wig and sat in the chair. After only a few moments, Marianne became very dizzy and sick to her stomach. I put her to bed. Mike finished the wig in another room.

There was just too much company, too many people and too much excitement for Marianne to tolerate. From now on, I am going to limit visitation to fifteen minutes per person.

Last night was a nightmare. Marianne threw up from the taste of something she ate. As she throws up, the pain is excruciating in her body. Why must she suffer like this? I keep praying, please God, take her pain away. I called the doctor. He told me to increase the number of pain pills. The doctor gave me a time formula to follow. Two pain pills every eight hours. Today, it will be 8 A.M. 4 P.M. and midnight.

Marianne is in terrible pain this Sunday morning. I am waiting to hear from Marianne's brother, Fred. He is coming to visit. Hopefully, Fred will help me find a few minutes of space each day to try to do some work. This terrible disease has cost me everything. The medicine is so expensive it's almost impossible to believe. Ten pills cost me $780. Yesterday, the pain medication cost $140. The additional medicine cost $130 more. By the way, the $270 medication doesn't seem to be working! I guess that's why it's called 'Practicing Medicine!' I'm sure today the doctor will change the medication and I'll buy more pills for practice. They will continue to practice until they come up with the right formula.

Marianne began hiccupping uncontrollably around 2 A.M. I got up and gave her the special hiccup pills. After about twenty minutes, she fell asleep. Again, around 4 A.M. the hiccups started. I gave her another pill. Around 4:30 A.M. she fell asleep.

January 21, 2001

Last night, it happened again. Hiccups throughout

the night. Yesterday, in spite of what I said about limited visitation, her girlfriend Sandra insisted on spending most of the day visiting Marianne. It was a mistake for me to allow such a long visit. The consequences were devastating. They consisted of another sleepless night for me, uncontrollable hiccups for Marianne and pain for her every time she would hiccup. This morning, we went to the Cancer Clinic. Dr. Allen injected Marianne s brain with more chemotherapy. She gave me two additional prescriptions, adding to the pile of pills that Marianne is already taking, about sixteen pills per day and night.

Marianne also got an injection to help her white count increase. It is very low. Dr. Allen told me that she was concerned about the quality of Marianne s life.

If God is going to grant my Marianne a miracle, now is the time. According to the doctor, her life is being extended by the chemotherapy, but the pain is increasing daily. I do not want Marianne to live in pain. Marianne and I talked about this at great length. My life, she said, is coming to an end. Once again she said, I am not afraid to die. I know I will be with God. She looked at me with those beautiful brown eyes, and said, Jerry I m so worried about you.

I told her how much I loved her and that I will always love her for the rest of my life. I couldn t help myself. I began to cry in front of her. Everyone has told me that I must be strong in front of Marianne and I know it s true, but I couldn t help myself. I held her close, being as gentle as possible. I whispered into her ear, Oh God, I love you, Marianne.

The nurse from the Nathan Adelson Hospice called

and made an appointment to meet at our house at nine o'clock tomorrow morning. She is going to fill me in on how they operate and will give me a breakdown on their assistance and care.

Marianne is very weak. I just gave her the pain medication she needs at four o'clock. Tonight, I will make her dinner and will serve her on the tray that I always try to make look nice. Usually, I put a flower on the tray. I cannot come to grips with the fact that I'm going to lose my Marianne. Life without her, is impossible for me to imagine. I do not believe that this is her time, no matter what. I will not change my mind.

I'm growing weaker every day, in so far as my ability to maintain the strength I need to stay awake all night, goes. During the daytime hours I take care of Marianne, by making sure that she has her medication on time, that she eats the right things throughout the day, etc.

I never leave her alone longer than a few minutes just to be sure that she's OK. The times that Marianne feels well enough to talk to me are like gold. We talk together, just like we used to, telling each other our thoughts, and always, in such wonderful honesty. Our doorbell just rang. Standing in the door were two mormon missionaries. They told me they received a call from Washington about Marianne and wanted to give her a blessing. I don't know how they knew her name and I have no idea who in Washington asked them to come to our house. We are not Mormons. In any event, Marianne is sleeping, so the blessing will have to wait.

I gave the two young missionaries our telephone number and they said they will call. I will accept this bless ing in the spirit in which these missionaries want to give it. I know Marianne will feel the same way I do, in this regard.

So far, we have had a Catholic Priest and a Jewish rabbi here at the house. The rabbi hung a Mezuzah on our front door and on our bedroom door. They have both prayed with Marianne. The priest gave Marianne a beautiful crucifix and he administered the last rights. Now, we will add the Mormons to the list. People all over the world are praying for Marianne. I continue to write letters to God, asking for a miracle. As crazy as it may sound, I have found that writing to God gives me a certain comfort, knowing that my prayers are etched on the paper, carrying my innermost thoughts.

January 22, 2001

Marianne was hiccupping all night, again. I gave her the medicine prescribed for hiccups but it simply does not work! Each time she hiccups, her entire body wretches forward, as if it is being catapulted into the air. I rubbed her back to try to soothe her. I talked to her all night, trying to keep her calm.

About 4 a.m. Marianne suddenly leaned on her elbow. She let out a loud rather long melodic kind of sound. It wasn't a scream, like the time she had the seizure, but it lasted much longer. It scared the hell out of me. I asked her what happened. "I heard loud noises in my ears," she said. "Oh, Jerry," she said. "It scared me!" I made her take two pills (seizure medicine) immediately. From that moment on, I sat in the chair watching her try to sleep, while she continued to have those horrible hiccups.

It is now 6 A.M. I have put the dishes in the dishwasher and cleaned the kitchen and the dining room. I fed the cat and the dog and took my high blood pressure medicine. Now, I will make breakfast for Marianne. I'll give her the medicine prescribed for morning and wait for the arrival of the nurse I spoke of earlier.

January 24, 2001

The worst day of all. Again, we were awake all night, as Marianne was uncontrollably hiccupping, unable to breathe properly. New medicine arrived tonight at 9 P.M. but all it seems to do is medicate Marianne, until she falls into a delirious stupor. Even in her sleep, she continues to hiccup.

The hospice nurses are coming every day. They have changed medications around and have found a way that isn't so confusing. Believe me when I tell you, there is a myriad of medications that must be given to Marianne. Marianne is in terrible pain. Mostly, the pain is in her head, behind her eyes. She is taking the most powerful pain medication, but still the pain persists.

Her brother, Fred and his wife Jan, have arrived. They are sleeping upstairs in my office. Our guest rooms are presently out of commission, filled with debris that Marianne has placed in these rooms over the past year. The rooms are simply out of bounds for everyone, including me. The nurses are trying to convince me that Marianne is dying quickly now and only has a short time left in this life. I don't care what anyone says. I still have a hope that God will grant a miracle or Marianne herself will rise above this monster called Small Cell Cancer and beat it. I simply can't come to grips with the thought of losing her. I never will. Never! If it comes to pass and I do lose my Marianne, I will have her inside of my heart, forever. I will never be without the memories of her love, her devotion, her intelligence, the incredible awareness, her gentle smile and most of all, her uncommon beauty.

Where did it all begin? The answer came from her older brothers and sister, whose memory of Marianne dated back to her birth date of June 12, 1950 in the St. Carolus Hospital, in Djakarta, Indonesia. Marianne was the youngest of four children; two brothers, John and Fred and her sister, Grace.

Her mother was devoted to Marianne and insisted on bathing her every day, even though she was busy with her daily responsibilities, overseeing many servants who, amongst other things, did laundry, dishes, made the beds and cleaned the fifteen room city house. Her mother also had the responsibility of overseeing their country estate located contiguous to their 500 acre rubber plantation.

Marianne's father, William Rhemrev, was not only the owner of a rubber plantation, he was also a teacher of agriculture. Unfortunately, the Japanese invasion of Indonesia turned everything around for the Rhemrev family. The Japanese took possession of all the property belonging to her father, William Vermeer Rhemrev including his plantation. The family was forced to flee to Holland on August 24, 1954.

They arrived in Maastricht, Holland and traveled to the town of Elshout, where they lived in an upscale immigration development. After approximately six months, they moved to Drunen Holland and into their own home. They remained in Drunen, until the family emmigrated to the United States. Their emmigration to America was sponsored by the Catholic Church. The family arrived in Woodburn, Oregon in 1961.

At that time, Marianne's older brother, Fred, was twenty-five years old. Her brother John, was twenty and her sister, Grace was twenty-one. Marianne was eleven years old and didn't speak a word of English. She was enrolled in Bolton Elementary School. Her brother, Fred, went to Oregon Poly Tech where he received an engineering degree. Marianne's brother, John, went to work for a large wholesale Import and Export Flower Brokerage firm and her sister, Grace, became a secretary for a local, law firm.

In 1963, the family moved to Oregon City. By the age of thirteen, Marianne had become a rare beauty. She was gorgeous and statuesque. As I said earlier, in spite of the fact that Marianne didn't speak a word of English when she arrived in America, she ended up to the top of her class one year later. I remember Marianne telling me that she learned to speak English by watching cartoons! I must admit, that didn't surprise me. As far as Marianne is concerned, nothing would surprise me. Today, her command of the English language is remarkable. Interestingly, though, when she gets upset with me, her words always come out in Dutch. Her telephone conversations with her family, who still live in Oregon, are mostly in Dutch.

Marianne graduated from Oregon City High School in 1969. She went to work for the Sheraton Hotel in Port land, Oregon as secretary to the general manager.

Wherever Marianne went, she was the center of the attention of every man in the area. Her beguiling beauty was amazing. Marianne began to get offers to represent certain products and pose in photographs representing them. Major manufacturing companies were after her. Among them were; Suzuki Motorcycle, Olympia Beer and Revlon. It was becoming obvious that a career as a model or an actress was at hand. Marianne felt the calling, but still hadn't made up her mind, as far as a career was concerned.

She met Stanley Marks in 1970. In a whirlwind courtship, against her father's advice, Marianne married Stanley Marks. But, the marriage was not to be. It lasted only six months. Marianne had made her decision. A quickie divorce from Stanley, who didn't understand what happened and a quicker trip to Hollywood, spelled out the end of her marriage, which was annulled, and the beginning of Marianne's show business career.

In no time, she was spotted by top Hollywood agents. Marianne went to acting schools and worked as a model, from time to time. She lived in a one bedroom apartment in west Los Angeles and maintained a rather low key, in as much as her social life was concerned. Marianne had a goal- to make it in Hollywood! Famous hair Magul, Vidal Sassoon, spotted her rare beauty. Marianne became his favorite, in-house, Hair Model. Playboy offered her centerfold exposure, but Marianne declined. She had other plans.

Laughingly, she told me that when she turned 50, she may decide to become a centerfold. Believe me, if

Marianne had made that decision, Playboy would have jumped at the chance. The acting schools finally paid off. Marianne received a co-starring role in a hit television series called *Fantasy Island*. From then on it, was downhill all the way. One show after the other. Marianne appeared on *Love Boat, Baretta, CHIPS* and other television series shows, until she was offered a co-starring role opposite Sean Connery in a Richard Brooks-film: *Wrong Is Right*. Marianne co-starred with Sam Elliot in an ABC Movie of the Week, *Wild Times*.

In 1988, she starred in the action adventure *Fists Of Steel* filmed on location in Hawaii. In Las Vegas, Marianne hosted countless television musical variety shows, game shows, talk shows, sporting events and institutional commercials.

She was the spokesperson for the state of Nevada's Motor Vehicle Division. Marianne won the New York Television Festival for best performance and best narration of the explosive documentary, *Get Madd*, the most comprehensive documentary ever produced on the subject of driving under the influence. During the past ten years, Marianne has been working hand in hand with me, to formulate and pre-produce the world's only high definition account, in live-action, of an audio-visual encyclopedia of the United States of America. Combining the money that we had earned over our twenty-three years of marriage, Marianne and I developed.

'*The United States of America Series*.' Our course was set. Marianne has achieved moderate success as an actress, great exposure and success as the spokesperson for countless Las Vegas Strip Hotel properties, through their institutional commercials. It is believed that through the combination of in-house commercials and other institutional commercials she has starred in or hosted, Marianne is seen around the world by approximately four million people each and every day. Everything in the outside world was now being put aside. We were living our lives, being completely devoted to our project or passion to produce this monumental, high definition, encyclopedic series of programs, to give to the world the first live-action, audio-visual encyclopedia, depicting more than 775 American cities, towns and rural areas and every capital city in the nation. Marianne has always wanted to be in a position to give to certain charities, her way! She has talked about this over the course of our marriage, on numerous occasions. I have always supported and liked the idea. Now, we have a project that can earn the kind of money that can make her dream come true.

With the sure-fire success of our United States of America Series, this would give Marianne that opportunity. It would, at the same time, fulfill my dream for her. I have always believed that Marianne's beauty and intelligence needs to be shared with the world.

This series will do that. It would cause her exposure to be monumental throughout the world, as the series has been set to be translated into thirty-one languages. It would also give her exposure to the American public for an unprecedented 156, continuous weeks. It must sound like this series was developed for the sake of causing Marianne to become a world wide success. It wasn't! We developed this series for our country. With the social and economic problems facing our nation's cities, towns and rural areas today the rest of the world is getting the wrong impression of our great nation. The production of *'The United States of America Series'* will demonstrate to the entire world, that this nation is, without question, the finest, most respectable nation in the world. That is our goal. That is why we packaged this property and have put most of our savings into it. Remember the man who said, "Ask not what your country can do for you, ask what you can do for your country?" To that end, we have developed this project.

Then, on August 3rd, the bottom fell out. Everything in our lives stopped. Everything had to be put on hold. As you have been reading, Marianne is fighting for her life. The doctors have given us one horror story after another. They began with, "Marianne won't live past the month of August 2001!" This is February, 2002 and the fight goes on. As I have continually said, I cannot believe that I will lose my Marianne. I understand that the doctors can only do so much. I also understand that they have given up. As it has been from the onset, Marianne's life is in the hands of God.

February 8, 2002

Marianne had a fair night. She was in pain yesterday and this morning, I had to give her three doses of the strongest pain medicine. She is having trouble remembering things; short term and long term. Strangely, though, from time to time, she remembers things that happened twenty years ago. The nurse just left, after examining Marianne. She told me that I was doing a good job with the medication. She advised me to take Marianne outside awhile, if she felt OK. She told me I could take her for a ride, if she's up to it. I walked the nurse outside. "Tell me," I said, "How's Marianne really doing." The nurse looked at me and took my hand.

"I'm sorry, Jerry," she said, "But Marianne is dying. Maybe it's not her time right now- today, but I can tell you from my experience, that it won't be that long!"

Oh God, I thought. Here we go again. These medical people have been putting Marianne into her grave since August 3 of last year. The other night, Marianne looked at me and said, "Honey, why do I have to die like this?" I told her that she's not going to die. "You're going to beat this thing, honey, I know you will." I was trying to give her hope. I was telling her how I felt. I was telling her what I wanted to happen, what I have been praying for every day and night. God knows I want her to live. Inside my heart, I'm not sure, anymore...

I'm so mixed up and confused about this killer disease. The doctors and nurses continue to give me their dialogue of hopelessness, which includes their constant suggestion that I put Marianne in the Hospice. I can guarantee there will be no chance of that ever happening. Marianne stays with me! No matter what!

February 9, 2002

Countless nights of no sleep have made me feel like I'm in a daze. I find myself staring at nothing, from time to time. Today, I mopped the kitchen floor, vacuumed, washed the dishes and cleaned the back yard. In between the chores I gave Marianne her breakfast and lunch and medicine at the times required. Bob Ahmanson is coming to visit tomorrow. Marianne is looking forward to seeing him.

February 10, 2002

The visit from Bob Ahmanson and his secretary, Fran, was really nice. Marianne got out of bed for the first time in three weeks and sat in the dining room, on the couch. Bob sat next to her and they ate lunch (box lunches that Bob and Fran brought from their jet). Marianne seemed happy. Thankfully she had no pain.

Bob and Fran stayed for an hour and a half, but had to leave for business reasons. We said our good-byes and Marianne went back to bed.

At around 5:30 P.M. Marianne walked into the kitchen. She found an empty tuna can that I had put some birthday candles in. She lined the candles up on her dinner tray. Red, blue, green, yellow, etc. After she lined them up she stood there and looked at the candles for quite a while. Then, she took the scotch tape roller and began to tape the candles to the inside of the tuna can. I didn't say a word. I just stood there and watched. After she taped all the candles to the inside of the can, she suddenly decided it wasn't right, so she removed them. Then, she spotted a small plastic cup and put the cup inside the tuna can. She began taping the candles to the inside of the plastic cup. Her expression was very serious, as though she was accomplishing something wonderful.

My God, I thought. *What is she doing?* But I still didn't say a word. I walked into the dining room and closed the sliding door that leads to our backyard and pool area. When I walked back into the kitchen, Marianne was gone! I felt a breeze. The front door was open. I walked to the front door and there was Marianne in our front yard, picking up rocks, and putting them into the cup filled with candles. I put my arms around her and helped her walk back inside. I must admit that the can with the candles and the rocks looks very artistic, but what else could one expect from Marianne? She put the small decorated can in the middle of a paper plate and quietly went back to bed.

The whole scene was surrealistic, to say the least. I will save the can. In fact, I put it on our coffee table.

February 10, 2001

Shar and Mike Tessario came to visit. Marianne loves Char. They talk for long periods of time. Marianne holds Char's hand. When Char visits, I leave them alone. Girl talk etc. I think it does Marianne good to visit with her friend alone. Sometimes, Mike stays in the room while the girls talk. After Char and Mike left, Melissa (another friend) came to visit Marianne. She also wanted to talk business with me. Melissa is a very ambitious, young lady, who is trying to get started in her own enterprise. Then, Shea came by and visited with Marianne. Shea is another business associate and friend, who has cooked several wonderful meals for Marianne. Shea offers lots of support at this trying time. Last night, Marianne slept until 4:45 A.M. I slept too. It was the most sleep I have had in twenty-one days/nights of tending to her. The sicker she gets, the more I love her. The weaker she becomes, the more I try to give her strength.

    Good days followed by bad days, seem to be the way of this thing. From time to time, Marianne gets into a dreamlike state. I know she is in pain, when she closes her eyes and lays on her side. In a crazy sort of way, when she gets like that, it seems to me that it's sort of a blessing from God. For those periods of time seem almost unreal, like she's floating in the twilight zone. Lately, her memory seems to be failing more. I guess that the correct analysis of what's happening right now is sort of a Cancerous Dance of Death! My Marianne is dying a slow, terrible death. I am doing everything I can to keep her out of pain and keep her in the best possible quality of life that I can provide. Sometimes, in a quiet moment, she looks at me and says things that break my heart. Two days ago, I was sitting on the floor next to the bed, holding her hand, telling her how much I love her. She looked at me with those big brown eyes and said, "Are you going to get married?" "My God Marianne what are you talking about?" I told her that I will never marry again. You ve got me forever honey, until the end of time! I kissed her cheek. That means forever! Is that OK with you? Marianne smiled. Yes, she said, it is but I want you to enjoy your life. Funny thing is, without Marianne I will have no life. She has been so much of an inspiration to me, so much of a part of me that words cannot express the empty feeling I get when I try to imagine what it would be like without her; without being able to hear her voice, or touch her hand or look at her beautiful face. I can t imagine what it would be like to come into our house and not find her home. Every time I come home the first thing I do is hug and kiss her. I ve done that for twenty-four years. I can t imagine life without my Marianne. I know I have my sons but they have their own lives to live. I love them and don t want to hurt them or my grandchildren but again, without Marianne what good is anything anymore for me.

February 11, 2002

Rosell Owens brought breakfast this morning. Every morning Rosell brings something for Marianne. Today he brought pancakes and fresh strawberries. He also brought some additional fresh fruit. As usual, I fixed Marianne a tray displaying the food so that it really looked as tempting as I could make it look. I added a cup of hot tea and served it to her in bed. She smiled a big smile and sat up fixing her pillows. It looked like she was going to eat for a change. I got her medicine and put it on her tray.

Don t forget to take your medication honey, I reminded her. She smiled and picked up the pills. Rosell sat in the chair and began talking with Marianne. Within a few short moments, Marianne began to throw up. Even though she hadn t eaten a bite of food, she got very sick to her stomach. Every day a new horror gets added to the equation. Yesterday she hiccupped throughout the day and couldn t eat. This morning it looks bad for the rest of the day as far as eating is concerned. I had to give her pain medication at 8 this morning.

February 14, Valentines Day

At 4 A.M. this morning, Marianne suddenly knocked everything off the small table sitting on her side of the bed. She got out of bed and went to the dresser, where I have placed twenty-four vials of medicine. For some reason, she began to take the bottles and place them in different areas on top of the dresser. When I spoke to her, she simply ignored me. She was tuned out (so to speak), which seemed to be the case. I think that the medication is taking its toll.

I called the nurse and asked if we could cut down on some of the medication. She said that tomorrow during her visit we could discuss cutting down. Marianne goes in and out of various stages of being awake. Sometimes, she s as sharp as ever, right on the money, but an instant, later she closes her eyes and goes off into oblivion. The nurse tells me that this is part of the course. I knelt next to Marianne s side of the bed and held her hand. When I looked at her beautiful face, I remembered a scene she did in a movie in 1988. Marianne was playing a Russian K.G.B. agent. The look on her face during that scene was the same as the look I see now. In the scene, Marianne was exchanging very serious dialogue with an actor, named Henry Silva. I wondered why that thought entered my mind at that moment. I knelt there, looking at her beautiful face. Again, tears started running down my face. I was in a state of utter disbelief. When I look at her beautiful face, Marianne seems almost unreal, like a porcelain doll. I know I ve said it before, but honest to God, Marianne seems like an angel, a real angel!

I haven t called Henry Silva to tell him what s going on with Marianne. We re friends and I owe him a call. The bedroom is filled with flowers, roses on top of roses. Bob Ahmanson sent Marianne a dozen red and the Sardelli family sent a dozen pink. The bar in our front room area is filled with flowers, sent by friends. Marianne has had such an active life, since we ve been married. It s been one show after another. In between shows, Marianne took care of every piece of business related to our company. No easy trick, since we had produced over seventy-eight television specials in two years. It was an unbelievable feat.

The feat was that Marianne starred in most of the shows. Not only that, she kept the books, made the payroll (sometimes as many as 125 people were on the payroll), never missed making dinner, doing the dishes, feeding the dogs and grooming them (at one time, we had three Pekinese and a Doberman pincher) and the list goes on. A remarkable girl, to say the least. I remember, from time to time, Marianne would look at me and say, You know honey, I can t eat that, because cancer runs in my family. Or, something would happen that would cause her to remind me about the fact that her family was riddled with cancer. I never believed that it would happen to Marianne. In fact just the opposite was always in my mind. How could a girl who works out every day, who never smoked or drank, who eats the best healthy food available, takes daily vitamins and generally took care of herself in an almost magical way get cancer? Not my Marianne. It couldn't happen to her. Obviously, I was wrong. It seems that nothing really matters. A person can do all the right things, but if that disease is in your destiny, your goose is cooked!

Through this nightmare, I'm starting to believe that there is a conspiracy at hand in the medical world. The treatments are superficial and, as I have said before, the doctors do a sort of paint by numbers routine, until they finally tell you that the chemotherapy isn't working anymore. Day by day, night by night, I watch my Marianne get weaker and weaker. I watch her lose the strength and power she always had. I watch her facial expressions that make my heart skip a beat, the sadness in her eyes, the hopelessness of it all. I try my best to keep her happy and most important, out of pain. I never leave her alone for more than a few, short minutes. I can't seem to be away from the bedroom, even when she sleeps.

February 15, 2002

This afternoon, the nurse from the Hospice came, at my request. I asked them to change the medicine from pills to liquid. Marianne is having a hard time taking so many pills. There are still two pills that have to be crushed or cut in half. The nurse asked me if I could cut a pill in half. I found my all-around knife with a 3" blade. I tried to cut the pill in half with it. It didn't work. Then, I took a fishing knife out of a drawer, but the nurse suggested that we crush the pills, instead. We ended up using an ice cream scooper as the crusher and a small, wooden bowl.

Bonnie Sax and her husband came over for a visit. As sick as she was, Marianne suddenly got out of bed just before they arrived and answered the door when they knocked. Bonnie was really surprised. So was I! Bonnie and Marianne went into the dining room area of our house and began to talk. Shelty and I went to the market. It was a chance for me to shop for the things I needed regarding the crushed pills etc. I had to buy applesauce to put the crushed pills in and fruit juice to disguise the liquid medicine etc...

When we returned from the store, Marianne and Bonnie were still in the dining room talking. I noticed a bunch of burned matches lying around the kitchen, but I didn't say anything about it at that time.

Marianne took the liquid at four o'clock. She didn't seem to have a problem. I crushed the pills as instructed and put them in some applesauce. Marianne ate it all.

This was the first time Marianne was out of bed for such a long time, almost two hours. We sat outside on our patio and ate fried chicken and potato salad with Bonnie and Shelty. The phone rang, as we were eating. It was the Hospice. The lady on the phone asked me about the knife I used to cut the pills! Then, she also asked about a gun! "What gun?" I asked. "There was no gun." I told her I used the knife to try to cut a pill in half. She told me that the Hospice has a rule about weapons. To be quite candid, the call was inappropriate and rather disconcerting, to say the least.. Then, about an hour later, the nurse called to ask about Marianne. I told her she was getting along fine. Then, she asked, "What about you? How are you doing?"

I told her I was OK. I asked her if I scared her with the knife I used to try to cut the pill in half. "No, she said. Frankly, I'm worried about you!" "What do you mean," I asked. "Well, she said, you don't have any help. We don't want to see you hurt yourself, when something happens to Marianne." I know these are Hospice people. Merchants of death, I call them. God knows they have helped me (I think) or, maybe they're part of the conspiracy I am starting to believe is very real, regarding cancer and health care, etc. The fact of the matter is, I can't understand why all of a sudden, the nurse seems worried about me and my state of mind!

I have never indicated anything to her or any of the members of that Hospice, that I would try to injure myself. I'm not suicidal. I told her that I loved my wife. All I want to do is care for her and help her. I said, "If I hurt myself, it would prevent me from doing that, wouldn't it?"

The nurse reminded me that I could bring Marianne into the Hospice. "You can stay there with her," she said. "No thank you, I said. We're not interested." From the onset these Hospice people have been telling me that I can bring Marianne into the Hospice. That is not what I intend to do.

Some years ago, Marianne and I talked about this kind of thing. We made an agreement, that if either of us were ever incapacitated, that the other would take care and we never would allow either of us to go into a rest home or a hospice. That was our deal. As I have indicated throughout this journal of events, Marianne and I have always had an honest relationship. We don't lie to each other. My marriage vow has never been violated and it never will. Till death do us part, is the deal. Marianne is comfortable in her own home. She is not going to a hospice or a hospital. We signed papers with the Hospice, at the onset of this nightmare. No heroics (as they call it), if something goes wrong. Marianne signed that paper. These people had better just take care of Marianne, like they agreed to do and forget about me. I'm not interested in their concern for anything, except my Marianne.

I told Bonnie and Shelty about the call. They couldn't believe it. They left about 4:30 P.M. Shea came over to visit Marianne about 5 P.M. Earlier today, we had a visit from my son Aaron's mother-in-law. A lovely, lady who said she wanted to help me out. Starting Monday the 18th she agreed to spend three hours with Marianne each day to give me a little relief. That will be wonderful. I have been caring for Marianne 24-7 since August 3, 2001. Three hours a day away, will give me a chance to try to get a show in line, go shopping without pressure or maybe give me a chance to just walk in the park for awhile.

February 16, 2002

Marianne slept very well last night. This morning,

around 4 A.M. she hiccuped a little, but thankfully, it stopped and she continued to sleep. Like I said, every morning since our last return from UCLA Medical Center, my friend, Rosell, has brought us breakfast. Meals on wheels, so to speak. When I try to pay, he won't accept the money. When Rosell is tied up, Clancy Rial brings the food. Once they were both busy, so they had Phyllis Paxton bring the food.

Me, Rosell, Clancy and Phyllis used to have breakfast every morning, before walking two miles in the park. We did it every day. Marianne would sleep in, because she use to stay awake most of the night, doing book work or cleaning the house.

During these trying times, I've learned a great lesson. As I care for my Marianne and I do the housework, it gives me a different perspective of just how hard Marianne has worked over the years of our marriage. My appreciation of her and the way she has cared for me is magnified thousands of times.

If I need shaving cream, I simply go to the cupboard and get it. If I want mouthwash, I open the drawer and there it is. My clothes are always clean, my socks and shorts are in the drawer, all folded properly. The fact of the matter is, I have been pampered by Marianne, the likes of which very few men could ever imagine.

Some years ago, we were producing a musical variety show, starring Debbie Reynolds. Marianne hosted the show. We shot it at the Imperial Palace Hotel, on the Las Vegas strip. Marianne and Debbie got along just fine. Marianne introduced Debbie and the other stars; Abbe Lane, Roger Miller, Doug Kershaw and Nancy Sinatra, during the show.

After the show, Marianne looked at me and smiled. "You know what, honey?" she asked, "I really enjoyed that. You are a great director."

"What do you mean?" I asked. Marianne and I have done more than fifty of these kind of shows in the past, but suddenly, I found Marianne saying she liked it. For some reason, she paid me a compliment. I don't mind saying, that I really liked being complimented by Marianne. It meant the world to me. For the most part, the shows represented great stress for both of us. I had to write them, budget the cost, produce, direct and cast the shows, while Marianne corrected my mistakes and helped guide me through every step of the production, including helping me set the venues for all the shows. On top of that, Marianne had to learn the dialogue I had written for her. That was usually done the night before the show or, even more unbelievable, on the way to the show in our car. That's right, Marianne is that good. She's that talented. Many times, we would shoot institutional commercials for Las Vegas strip hotels. I would arrange the production, but I wouldn't write one word of dialogue for Marianne. I would simply set up the scenes for Marianne and she would wing it. Interestingly, she always gave the right information about whatever area of the hotel she was taking about. It didn't matter if it was a restaurant, the coffee shop, the shops and stores in the hotel or, for that matter, the casino. Marianne could tell you the odds on every game! When we produced Ralph Engelstad's antique & classic auto collection video (known as one of the best antique collections in the world), Marianne committed to her memory the makes, cost, year of manufacture and other information about more than fifty of the great machines in the collection.

As usual, Marianne was beautiful and delightful in the video. Many people told me that they had a hard time looking at the cars, when Marianne spoke or demonstrated things, like articulated headlights on one of the fabulous, antique cars. Her presence on film has always amazed me. She has the voice of an angel and a face that is exquisite. She is quite beautiful and stately. Many times, her exotic beauty worked as some kind of deterrent in the business. Certain male and female actors were jealous of Marianne's beauty and didn't want to be in scenes with her. Sounds silly, but it happens to be true, especially if you know actors. Sean Connery didn't mind, but he has worked with beautiful, exotic women all of his career. Neither did Sam Elliot or Sammy Davis or Marie Osmond and countless other stars, who loved working with Marianne. But, there was that strange under current of jealousy that I recognized, but couldn't do anything about.

February 17, 2002

Another sleepless night for, me as Marianne had those horrifying hiccups all night long. Thankfully, they stopped about 5 A.M. It started to get light outside, so I just forgot about sleeping. Marianne ate a huge breakfast. She took all of her medication, with only a small battle about one of the new drinks of medicine that she has decided she doesn't like. I changed the patch, which is preventing pain (so they say) and Marianne fell asleep.

My son, Aaron came over this morning with my granddaughter, Sydney. Sydney checked on Marianne, to see if she was sleeping, as Aaron worked on my computer. Thank God, Marianne seems to be resting comfortably, with no pain.

February 18, 2002

Marianne stopped taking her medicine yesterday. She also stopped eating and drinking. After the great breakfast on the morning of the 17th, she seemed to shut down, not wanting anything at all. I spent the entire day in the bedroom with her. She has stopped talking. She simply cannot talk. Marianne seems to be falling into a coma. She reacts when I kiss her, but she has not uttered a word since the 17th.

I stayed awake most of the night, holding Marianne close and telling her how much I love her. Even though there was no response, I know she can hear me and I know she knows how much I adore her.

Char and Mike came over. Char sat with Marianne for quite a while. Even Char couldn't get Marianne to acknowledge her presence.

February 19, 2002

Again, I held Marianne close all night. I know that she is dying now, for sure. I can feel her life-force leaving her body. I can see the empty look in her beautiful eyes, as she stares into oblivion. Her eyes are open, but I know she cannot see. The cancer has caused Marianne to go blind. She has taken no food or drink or medication for almost three days and nights, now.

Jack Snyder, from the Nevada Highway Patrol, came over this afternoon, to spend some time. He brought me a hamburger, which was great, since I haven't eaten today. Allen Young and Jeep Capone's wife visited today. Kathie watched Marianne, while Al and I went to the store to buy some Simple Green, so I could mop the floors. Upon our return, Marianne still remained almost unconscious. She opens her eyes but, as I said, they seem empty. Her silence is deafening to me. I want so much to hear her beautiful voice. I went looking for a candle. I don't know where anything is in this house, except for my computer, the bedroom , bathroom and shower. I write, eat, sleep, produce shows and love Marianne. That's my life. While I was looking for the candle, I came across a small book that had a tiny little padlock on it. Curiosity killed the cat. I opened the lock, by breaking it open. I discovered notes written by my Marianne, sort of a journal. I am going to share some of those notes with you, so you will get the picture of just how wonderful and saintly Marianne really is.

MARIANNE S NOTES:

Wednesday - April 26, 2000 - 9 p.m.

I thank God for my wonderful husband who loves me and who takes care of me to the very best of his ability.

I am thankful for my love & caring for him as I cannot think of anyone else I would rather love and take care of.

I am thankful for friends like Beth Blackburn to whom I can be of assistance to her in her life decisions. It gives me a sense of worthiness in this life. I am also thankful to have Beth just to talk to as "girls do"

I am thankful for people in business like Richard Lo Presto who is always kind + 85% happy. I am thankful that I am able to assist him in viewing alternative perspectives on various business & personal situations.
I appreciate that he is mindful of God and that he openly speaks of God & spirituality.
I am thankful for the chicken caesar salad he brought to me.

I am thankful for living in a beautiful home which I enjoy everyday.

I am thankful for my beautiful and fragrant garden

and swimming pool & my magic forest for the magic forest is my daily reminder that there is a living & true God who watches over us and all that we do...
9:20 p.m.

1:45 a.m April 28, 2000

I am grateful for my health and my body which has served me well.

I am grateful for the ability and the time I took this day to exercise physically from
2:15 p.m. to 2:45 p.m. (30 minutes) + from 3:19 p.m. to 4:16 p.m. (almost 1 hour) for a total of approximately one and half hours of aerobics and fifteen minutes of upper body + 370 crunches.

I am grateful for the wonderful food I ate this day. Also grateful for my ability to create tasteful dinners.

I am grateful that we have enough money for me to go to the grocery store and purchase whatever we like.

I am grateful that we have enough money for me to purchase food to help Martin and Curtiss who live next door and who are struggling in many areas of their lives.

I thank God that he has blessed Jerry and I with another beautiful day.

April 28, 2000 Friday

I am grateful for sharing a wonderful dinner with my husband and also with Lou and Mary Tabat at the Yukon Grill Restaurant celebrating Lou's 77th birthday.

I am grateful that I look good and that I have nice clothes that fit well.

April 29, 2000 - Saturday
I am grateful that our dog Banner is behaving so well in the house and does not upset anything.

I am grateful for the cookie samples from Smiths Market.

I am grateful for being able to do my aerobic exercise today (50 minutes with effort).

I thank God that he has kept us safely this day.

April 30, 2000 - Sunday

I am grateful for this day as it holds the promise of getting the finance for our USA Series. It is the most important thing for Jerry that he wants to accomplish. He wants to do this more than anything...I hope and pray that this will happen too. I have made my main (and only) effort in life to assist Jerry in his endeavors—to the exclusion of any career that I wanted to pur sue—when we get the finance and then complete the Series I will be able to do things of good will for many many people who truly need food and shelter—I believe that this is my calling in life. I don't know exactly how I will go about doing it but when the time comes I will get enlightened and God will send me a helper(s).

The fame and glory this series will crate will be useful for my ultimate goal, as mentioned. I hope and pray that my goal will become a reality—there are so many people who need just the basic necessities of life.

Please God let me help them. I am only able to do small things now.

May 1, 2000 - Monday

I am grateful for my kind and loving husband.

I am grateful that Sandy Dobritch is attempting to assist us re: the finance of the movie Jerry wrote for me along with other projects.

I am grateful that God gave me creative talents in the culinary department as Jerry loved my salmon dinner.

I am grateful for the gorgeous weather and beautiful outdoors we have and also our "magic forest" is more beautiful then ever.

I am grateful for being a blessed child of God.

Thank you God for watching over us. We need you to please keep us from harm.

Thank you Opa & Oma & Dad & Mom S. & Nana for being with us. Thank you Gene Toll for having chosen to be one of my spirit guides. Thank you all for assisting Jerry and me in what we are trying to do...please help us keep out of harms way...please know we appreciate that you are with us each day.

May 1, 2000 - Monday

I am grateful for God's goodness and abundance in my life.

I am grateful that he has made Jerry's eyesight come to more or less normal.

I am grateful for our good health.

May 4, 2000 - Thursday

I am grateful for the beautiful summer spread I have on our bed.

I am grateful that I was able to call 1-800 Now Pray, and have Jerry and I put on the prayer list for the next 30 days. Thank you God for all of your wonderful gifts— Please Lord, please send some luck our way we really need some luck to get our projects on the way.

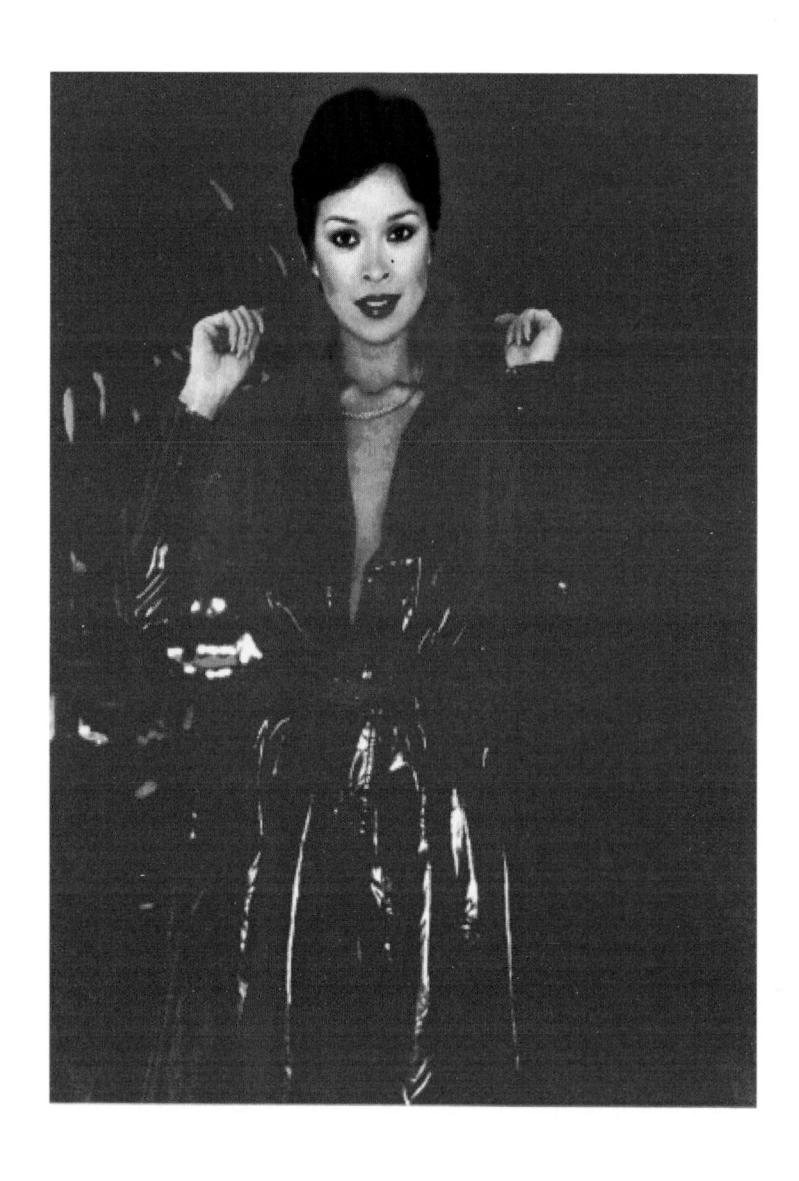

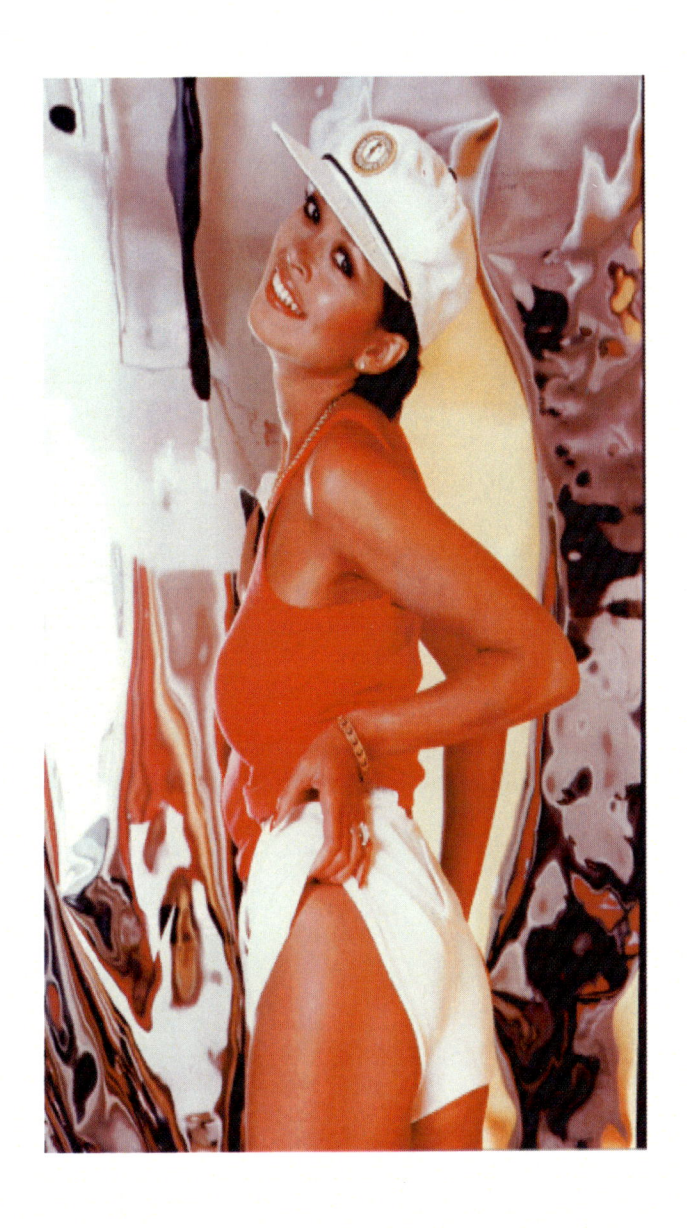

These are just a few of the entries in Marianne's journal. Hopefully, it will give you a pretty good picture of just who this girl I am writing about really is, along with her love of God. All Marianne ever wanted to do in her life with me, was to have a big enough hit to make enough money to help the homeless, and help underprivileged and neglected children. Like I said earlier, we both know that our America series will do just that, but God has not seen fit to let that happen…yet! I feel it is my obligation to get this series produced, so that I can dedicate it to the memory of Marianne and etch her name into history, until the end of time. That will be all I will work for, for the rest of my life. I must find a way to get it on.

February 20, 2002

I remained awake all night, again. Marianne is still not moving much at all. She can move her arms, but not her legs. She cannot speak, eat, drink or talk.

From time, to time she makes frightening sounds, that lead me to believe that she is in pain. I wash her face with a warm washcloth and try to moisten her lips several times each hour. Seeing her go through this, has changed my way of thinking about life, death and the medical profession. How can I relate the heartbreaking twenty-four hours a day death watch, I am presently doing with my Marianne. To see my beautiful, stately, gorgeous wife lying there completely helpless, is tearing my heart out. She is so brave and her soul so powerful, that even in this state, it must be uncommon to see the way she is hanging on to her life.

At 3:00 A.M. this morning, I talked to Marianne and didn't stop talking until after 4:00 A.M. I told her my thoughts regarding her wonderful contribution to our marriage and to me, personally. I told her that she was the smartest, most beautiful, giving, loving, talented person I have every had the privilege of knowing. I told her that I would love her through eternity. And I will! Marianne has made an indelible mark on my heart. I told her I was writing this book about her life's experiences and gave her many of the details. I talked to her about how I had learned how her family emmigrated from Indonesia to Holland and later, to America. I explained how I found the right dates and times, by talking with members of her family in Oregon and in Amsterdam. I moved close to her and whispered into her ear. I said, "You know something honey. You are special, very special. Not just special to me, honey. You are an Angel! I mean, a real, honest to God, Angel." As I whispered to her, there was no expression on her beautiful face, but I could tell she was hearing me. It gave me a sense of accomplishment, in the strangest kind of way. I also told her that I know she will be getting wings and will be able to fly anywhere in the world, as long as she wants to. Incidentally, I really believe that! I know its true.

The nurses arrived at noon today. After their examination of Marianne they asked me to sit in the dining room, saying they needed to speak with me. They informed me that, in their opinion, Marianne is dying now and will not live too much longer. "Have you made funeral arrangements?" the nurse asked? I began to cry. "No, I haven't I said... I'm not sure how to do it." The nurse agreed to help me. "What do you want to do?" she asked. Marianne and I want to be cremated. We want our ashes to be put into the Pacific Ocean. The cremation will take place in Las Vegas. I will take Marianne's remains to Los Angeles and take her out to sea and cast her ashes into the ocean. I know for sure that her soul will be in heaven very quickly and she will be in the House of the Lord. I know that she will find it to be just like she has always imagined, only better…much better!

Tomorrow, I will continue with the arrangements for the church, because I know that Marianne wouldn't want her service to take place in a mortuary. I will arrange a dignified service, with a Catholic priest. I will put up a magnificent photograph of Marianne, so everyone can remember how radiant and beautiful she is.

I say 'is,' because as far as I am concerned, my Marianne will never be 'was.' She will always be alive, inside my heart forever.

February 21, 2001

Needless to say, I spent a very nervous night. My son, Aaron, stayed the night, to give me some support. I am truly thankful for it at this time. Being alone is difficult, at a time like this. Aaron and I were in the bedroom at the same time last night, watching Marianne sleep. We could see her eyes open, from time to time and we took turns talking to her.

After awhile, I got a washcloth and wiped her face off. I tried to drip a little water into her mouth. It seems so dry. Suddenly, both Aaron and I were on our knees kneeling next to the bed. We both began to cry. Seeing Marianne in this condition is so heartbreaking, I find it almost impossible to find the words to describe how it really was. As Aaron walked out of the bedroom, he turned to me and said, "Dad, if you need me, I'll be in the other room."

I got into the bed and positioned myself, so that I was able to touch her, without disturbing her sleep. Marianne slept through the night, with no incidents. She continually made a loud guttural sort of sound, but no more hiccups. She is unable to move at all. She just lays on her back, with her head on the pillow, waiting to be taken. Even though Marianne can no longer speak, I have spent lots of time talking to her, telling her that it's OK to go on to her next adventure. I have assured her that I will be joining her and we will be together for eternity. Inside I knew it was important for me to let her know it was OK for her to go.

I stayed awake looking at her, watching her sleep, remembering the many wonderful times we had together during our marriage. During the years of our marriage, I have told Marianne many times that there was no place on earth that I would rather be, than at home with her, alone in our house. Not the greatest restaurant in the world, nor the finest show or anything else, could take the place of just being alone with her.

That's the way I have always felt about being with Marianne. Now, all I can do is make sure that I am holding her, as she goes off to her new adventure and pray that I will be with her for eternity, when I die.

February 21, 2002

Marianne is looking worse. She lay awake all night last night, with her eyes wide open, trying desperately to breathe. The sound is raspy, like she's trying to clear her throat. I am going to call my sons and ask them to come home as soon as possible. Mark is in New York. Erik is in Taiwan and Morgan is in California. I told the boys that Marianne was dying. I asked them to come. Morgan arrived later that afternoon. Mark arrived in the evening and Erik, who had to fly from Taiwan, arrived on the 22nd. The boys were visibly shocked to see little Marianne lying there, unable to speak, her eyes wide open, but unable to see and the raspy breathing sound seemed to be growing louder with each breath she took. The boys took turns speaking to Marianne. I watched each of them kiss her on the cheek and on her forehead. They were crying. After that, they took turns, one at a time, being alone with my Marianne. They knew her time was short and they wanted to say goodbye in their own way, in privacy.

I have spent countless, sleepless nights watching Marianne, listening to her take one painful breath after another and feeling my heart sadden more and more with each breath.

February 23, 2002

I spoke with Marianne in desperate anticipation of what I knew was about to happen. I wanted to be sure she knew exactly how I felt even though I must have repeated it a hundred times over the past few days. I reiterated how much I loved her. I told her how grateful I was to God for having been allowed to spend the time we had together. It now appeared that Marianne was in pain. She was perspiring profusely. I continued to wipe her little face with a cool wash rag all through the night. I was getting desperate. I called the hospice at 6:30 A.M. and asked for a nurse to come as soon as possible. I could tell that Marianne was now in her last minutes of life and I was about to lose my dearest friend and the love of my life. I began to cry uncontrollably, as I knelt next to her, holding her hand. I spoke to her, repeating myself over, and over again. I continued telling her how much I loved her. I assured her that it was OK for her to go to God. I told her again and again, that I will be joining her, as soon as my time comes. Marianne couldn't move. She seemed paralyzed. I continued wiping off her face and putting mouth wash on a small swab inside her mouth.

The nurse arrived. He put his stethoscope against Marianne's chest. He looked at me, shaking his head. "I'm sorry Jerry," he said, "But your wife is dying." I called out to my boys. They ran into the bedroom and surrounded the bed. I knelt next to Marianne, so that I could touch her shoulder and her face with my left hand. Mark was next to me, holding my right hand. Erik stood next to Mark and Morgan was standing next to him. The nurse was standing at Morgan's left.

Marianne was desperately trying to breathe. She was gasping for air. I began talking to God, asking him to take my Marianne. Again, I told Marianne that it was OK to go. I couldn't stop crying, as I spoke. Oh, God, I love you Marianne. I reached up and kissed her cheek, as she drew her last breath.

At 7:54 A.M., Marianne was pronounced dead. I was in a state of indescribable shock. I held her hand and the boys just stood there, stunned. One at a time, they came over and kissed Marianne goodbye. The boys left the room. I continued talking to Marianne. In death, she was still as beautiful as ever. My God, how she fought this horrifying disease.

Never one time, through all of the trials and tribulations of the ordeal in the hospitals, at the Cancer Clinic or in the doctors office, did she ever complain. She was the bravest, strongest, most wonderful girl that God ever put on this earth. I am heartbroken beyond description. I feel that my life is also over without Marianne.

My boys are trying to comfort me, while at the same time, they immediately, began to pitch in to help me organize. Mark and Morgan took the bull by the horns. They are the oldest and they knew that Marianne was in complete control of our finances, both personal and for our company. They also know that I am not domesticated, having never paid a bill of any kind for twenty-five years. Marianne did it all. As a consequence, I can't find anything, not even our checkbooks.

I am in a daze now. I'm trying to go along with the boys, but my heart is so broken, that I can't think straight. My mind keeps whirling with thoughts of the past seven months. My God, Marianne tried to fight this small cell cancer, but in retrospect, I know beyond the shadow of a doubt, that she did it for me.I remember back when she was diagnosed with the disease and how she immediately, told me that she did not want chemotherapy. I remembered how she looked, as she told me that. The look on her beautiful face was one of resolve. Marianne knew exactly what she wanted to do or should I say, what she didn't want to do! I remember her saying "Let God take me, Jerry. I feel honored that he wants me and I'm ready to go!"

I was resolved to her will. I had made up my mind that it was her life and it was my responsibility to support her, no matter what. As I have written, when we arrived at UCLA, for some reason, Marianne changed her mind. She looked at Dr. Rosen, after he explained that he could extend her life and possibly put the cancer into remission. She said, "OK, Doc, lets give it a try." And God knows, she tried.

As I have also said, when Marianne made the decision to take chemotherapy, I didn't say a word. I sat next to her to support her, but I didn't open my mouth or make any suggestions. As I have said, I know now, beyond the shadow of a doubt, that Marianne decided to take chemotherapy for me. She did it for me!

As a result, Marianne suffered seven months of indescribable pain and humiliation during the treatment and series of tests she was subjected to at the UCLA Medical Center and the cancer clinic. I know that Marianne knew from the onset it was a hopeless case. I also know that her love for me was stronger then any pain she suffered or any humiliation she endured for seven torturous months. As I remember these things, I also remember that when Marianne was dying, I touched her cheek and began to pray. I prayed aloud. Please, God, when my time comes, let me be with my Marianne for eternity."

Marianne's funeral was held at St. Viator Roman Catholic Church at 1 o'clock in the afternoon on Thursday, February 28, 2002. There were approximately one hundred fifty people in attendance including Las Vegas hotel owners, many law enforcement personnel from the Nevada Highway Patrol and the Las Vegas Metropolitan Police Department. These were police officers who knew Marianne, having worked with her in a variety of documentary programs she hosted regarding their departments. Bob Ahmanson and Fran flew in from Los Angeles and were sitting next to me during the services. My cousin Joanie and her husband Neil also flew in from Los Angeles. Many more of our good friends from California were there, including Bruce Cash who has been very supportive of me through this whole ordeal. My close friend Nelson Sardelli delivered a beautiful eulogy. Everyone in the church was crying as he spoke. I have known Nelson since 1964. He has been a close friend of mine and Marianne's.

After the church services everyone was invited to the Imperial Palace Hotel where the owner, Ralph Engelstad and his general manager Ed Crispell arranged for coffee and snacks for everyone. It took place in the hotel Royal Hall C. As a special attraction Ed Crispell arranged through the hotel's advertising department to provide two large television screens and displayed a program depicting many of Marianne's starring and co-starring roles during her lifetime. Before I went to the hotel, I had the limo driver take me home so I could put Marianne's remains on our mantel. I began talking to her.

I told her where I was going. I gently placed the urn on the mantel, then said, "I love you, honey." I walked out the door crying, with a broken heart.

When I arrived at the hotel, it was hard for me to compose myself, before going into the royal hall. There was a large sign in front of the door that simply said 'SCHAFER' Mostly everyone from the church was there. It was a sad affair. These things always are. But the fact that the hotel had provided the large screen television sets and people could see Marianne's beautiful face and hear her voice made things seem a little better. People were talking in various groups. As I looked around, I noticed that during every conversation in every group, the folks kept looking away, focusing their attention on the two big television screens, where my Marianne was doing her thing.

My friend, Bruce Cash, walked over to me and handed me a paper. Here, he said. "I wrote this poem for Marianne."

MARIANNE'S POEM

(Never Far, Always Near)
Never Far
As we both knew, And you held me
Whispering, I love you!
Always Near
I will always be,
Do you hear God calling to me
Never Far
Will you ever be
From My Heart
Always Near
We have always been,
As even now, we are not apart
Never Far

Have we been from the other,
or will I now be from you
Always Near
Blowing kisses, Softly
Fluttering and Always True
Never Far
Are we from Heavens Gate
As the Angel, does patiently wait
Always Near
God does stand, As I reach and take his hand
And he holds me, As we walk together to the Promised land.

Once again, a friend displays how Marianne touched their hearts. She was a beautiful asset to this world. I remember when I first met her, I wrote her a note that said, "In this world of ordinary people, I'm glad there is you!" Marianne framed that note and it hangs in our house to this day, 25 years later.

March 8, 2002

These past few days have been like a mirage to me. I can't seem to function. It isn't getting easier. It's getting harder for me without Marianne. I remember her telling me once that if anything should happen to her, it would take five people to do what she does. As the days go by, I realize, once again, how right she was. Five won't be enough!

Bonnie Sax and her husband Shelty have asked me to go to the Venetian Hotel to watch their daughter Melinda perform. Although I am not really ready to go into a showroom, I feel that their friendship warrants a little effort on my part.

They picked me up around 6:00 P.M. We drove to the hotel. We met with Moti Shipara and a group of his friends, which included five girls from Argentina, who were visiting Las Vegas. Our party consisted of nine people.

By the time the show ended, I was beat to a frazzle. All I wanted to do, was to go home to be with my Marianne. I know it sounds crazy, but to me, she's still there. Suddenly, Melinda, the star of the show, stepped out on stage and announced that her mother was in the

audience. She also told the audience that the show they had just seen, was dedicated to Marianne Schafer, who was a close friend of her mother's. Bonnie stepped up on the stage and read this to the audience:
She read:

"This is for my friend Marianne"
A friend came into my life
one that I once knew
She said you look familiar
I smiled because I knew
It wasn't in this lifetime
But in another way before
its simple we had passed through the ongoing swinging door.
She kept comparing me to friends
she thought looked somewhat like me
I laughed within myself because I could already see. I recognized her spirit. It was like a bright and shinning star
and I will always find her she will never be too far.
She has the courage of a General and the strength of a roaring Lion.
I know we will always meet time after time.
We will see each other often we'll meet in some strange place
and once again she'll say to me you have a familiar face
And this time I will tell her cut it out Marianne,
We'll go down this road together again and then again.
God's light will shine on her today and one thing is for certain

she will never go away not even with the final curtain.
Someday when my light goes out I already know that I will always find her I'll just look for the brightest glow.

I looked around the audience and saw many people crying. Naturally I was one of them. It was wonderful of Bonnie to have her daughter dedicate the show to Marianne.

March 9, 2002

At 9 A.M. this morning, Bob Ahmanson is picking me up to fly me to Long Beach California, where we will take a boat out to sea and I will scatter Marianne's remains. I will put her favorite crucifix with her, the one that Sam Fisher bought her in Mexico. For me, this will be the beginning of trying to live my life without my Marianne. Oh, I know the old adage, life goes on…but for me, it is quite different. Marianne and I were inseparable, during twenty-five years of being together twenty-four hours a day. As I have said we worked for eleven years on a project called '*The United States Of America Series.*' As I have also said, I feel it is my obligation to my Marianne to cause this project to achieve its finance and dedicate the production to the memory of Marianne Schafer, without whose work, advice and creative contributions, this project would never have happened.

If I am successful, the screen will light up with

MARIANNE MARKS SCHAFER PRESENTS THE UNITED STATES OF AMERICA SERIES
and Marianne's photograph will be superimposed over the entire screen. This will place my Marianne into history, until the end of time. *'The United States of America Series'* is the first Live Action Audio-Visual Encyclopedia ever produced of our nation. It will be released around the world in thirty-one languages and will become a historical teaching tool in schools around the world. It will also be a masterpiece home entertainment series, containing thirty-two hours of encyclopedic information, depicted in High Definition Television.

It will provide information about 775 American cities, towns and rural areas and every capital city in the nation. As I have written, this has been our dream. We have worked for eleven years to assemble the information necessary and to create the proper materials and technical support to cause this to become a reality. Marianne even invented new words that I'm sure will be put into the dictionary. As an example, 'EDUTAINMENT.' You see, our series is a combination of entertainment and education, so Marianne coined 'EDUTAINMENT,' That's not all she did. During these 11 years, we spent most of our savings on preparation for this series. We have no partners. We paid all the costs ourselves. Marianne's insight was my biggest help. She had an uncanny way of being able to almost foresee the future. Through her insight, I could eliminate potential sponsors, who I had targeted to see. "I wouldn't waste my time with them. She'd tell me, they are not right for our project." That was all it took! If Marianne said no it was 100% of the time the right decision.

Flying to California with Marianne in the urn won't be easy. I can't stop thinking about it. I'm trying to tell myself that when I put Marianne's remains into the sea, it will be a new beginning for us both. I have to go on and try to do the America Series because I know that's what Marianne would want me to do. I also know that I will have to wait for God to take me in order to be with Marianne again. I still have the same incentive. I'm doing it for my Marianne. She is my guiding light, she always has been. As far as I am concerned she always will be. I will continue writing after I put her ashes into the ocean. I will, that is, if I can relax enough to be creative the way Marianne wants me to be.

At 9 A.M. Bob Ahmanson landed at the Executive Terminal in Las Vegas. He flew us to Long Beach, California. I held the urn containing Marianne's remains on my lap during the entire flight. I prayed to God to bless Marianne and to love her and welcome her into his house. Bob Ahmanson had already arranged to have a limousine waiting at the airport. The driver drove us to a place called Rocky Point, King Harbor, located in Redondo Beach, California. The ride took about thirty minutes. I found myself holding the urn tighter, and tighter as we got closer and closer to our destination.

At the marina, we were met by the captain of the ship. He was dressed in a suit and tie, not what I expected at all. I had visions of a fellow wearing a sea captain's cap, with white sneakers and white pants, etc., but no, this captain was different.

As I boarded the boat, the captain asked me to hand

the urn to him. He told us he would return in a few minutes and he disappeared below deck. Bob Ahmanson, his secretary, Fran and Shelty Matarazzo were on the boat with me. Shelty flew with me from Las Vegas, to keep me company and to offer support. God knows I needed it.

A few minutes later, the captain appeared, carrying a beautiful, white basket, filled with white carnations, surrounded by greenery. He told us that he had removed Marianne's remains from the urn and had placed them in the basket. Attached to the basket was a white rope. The captain explained that once we got out to sea, he would say a few words and then he would put the basket over the side and gently set it in the ocean. Then, he said, "I will take this hook and put it around the handle of the basket. That will turn the basket over."

He looked at me and quietly said, "At that point, Mr. Schafer, your wife's remains will be scattered into the ocean."

As we headed out to sea, I held the remains of my Marianne close to my chest, silently repeating my prayer to God to take Marianne into his loving arms. Finally, we reached our destination, west longitude 11850.05 North latitude 335006. As the boat bobbled in the water, the sound of the waves hitting the sides of the boat was the only sound I could hear. My mind was whirling with thoughts of my Marianne. I felt quite empty inside. I wanted to die. The captain stepped forward and said, "This time and place has been chosen to honor the life of Marianne Schafer. Soon, after each of us entered, we become aware of our world around us. We become aware of birth and of life and soon, we know of death. Even though we are well aware of death as a part of life, we find that the experience of death is never easy.

"As we continue in life, we find that nature has ways of helping us with our grief. Memories of the past become important to us. The love and personal experience we have shared, comes to memory quite often. Knowing of the peace that comes to those who go before us, seems to help. Nature has a way of helping."

The captain began to read from a small book. "Do not stand at my grave and weep. I am not there. I do not sleep. I am a thousand winds that blow, I am the diamond's glint on snow. I am the sunlight on ripened grain. I am the gentle autumn's rain.

"When you awaken in the mornings hush, I am the swift, uplifting rush of quiet birds in circled flight. I am the soft stars that shine at night. Do not stand at my grave and cry. I am not there, I did not die."

Then, the captain said, "As we prepare to place the earthly remains into the sea and return her body to the beauty of nature, shall we perform this duty in the spirit of love, honor and affection. Shall we be thankful for all of the goodness in life and allow the spirit to be free in the greatness of nature. We ask for the blessings upon each of us, as we move ahead into life with wonderful memories."

Tears were running down my face, as the captain stepped in front of me and asked me to hand him the basket. As I handed it to him, it seemed like my heart stopped beating. The captain placed the basket into the ocean. The basket began to float out to sea. After a few moments, the captain took a large hook and placed it over the handle of the basket. Then, he gently turned it over. I watched Marianne's remains scatter into the sea. At first, I felt heartbroken. Tears welled up in my eyes and I began to cry. I looked at Bob Ahmanson and he was crying, too. So were Shelty and Fran.

I threw one of the flowers the captain had given me into the ocean and at that moment, I realized that I had put my Marianne into the most powerful place in the world! After all, the ocean is nothing but power and life and constant movement. It is clean and beautiful and now, it is even more beautiful because it has accepted my beautiful Marianne.

The sun was reflecting on the ocean, as the captain started the boat and headed back to his slip in the marina. I kept looking at the ocean, reflecting light patterns from the sun, which magnified my earlier feelings that Marianne was truly in the best place she could be-in Heaven, of course.

As we drove back toward the airport, Bob, Shelty and I rode in the back seat. Fran sat up front with the driver. I looked at Bob sitting next to me. I could feel his grief. He has been so supportive during these past months. I will be eternally grateful. Something told me to give Bob the urn. I looked at him and said, "Here, Bob." I handed him the urn. "I want you to have this!" Bob began to cry. He held the Urn close to his chest and kissed it.

As the limousine continued toward the airport my mind was whirling. I was remembering the past seven months in fast forward time. The horrifying chemotherapy sessions and the other tests the doctors insisted on giving Marianne. The way Marianne never once complained, even through horrifying pain and suffering. I remembered her smiling face, her beguiling beauty, the softness of her skin, her white teeth, her beautiful hair. Her hands looked like those of an angel. I remembered her dying breath and the futility of it all. Oh my God, why did she have to go so young, why? I cannot say Goodbye to my Marianne or kiss her again or hold her hand or tell her I love her or see her smile or listen to the sound of her beautiful voice.

    I remembered after she passed away and everyone left the room, how I continued to talk to her. Once again, I found myself telling my Marianne that I would be with her in eternity. Over and over, I told her how much I loved her and for the last time, I kissed her goodbye.

HOW DO I SAY GOODBYE?

*Of all the words I've said in my lifetime
some were happy, some made me cry
but the hardest words for me to say are,
Goodbye
How do I say goodbye to someone I love this way
to the only one I've ever known
I love in every way.
How do I say goodbye to truth and love and hope
words just won't come to me
they're caught stuck in my throat
How do I say goodbye to a girl like Marianne
who has been my inspiration and my life.
How do I say goodbye to a girl like Marianne
who has shared every moment as my wife.
Marianne I will always love you
till the last day of my life
and when I die we will be together
and share eternity forever
Goodbye for now Marianne, Goodbye My Marianne, Goodbye.*

    Now it's time to talk about Marianne's life. When Marianne was nineteen years old, she became Miss Portland Oregon. A few months later, unbeknownst to anyone in her family, including her husband of six months, she left Oregon and drove to Hollywood, California to explore her dream. She had decided to become an actress! A model! Maybe even a Star. Marianne had no friends in Hollywood. In fact, she didn't know a soul.

    She had a few hundred dollars in her pocket that she saved, working as a secretary for the General Manager of the Sheraton Hotel in Portland. When she left Oregon, she didn't take anything from her husband Stanley Marks, except his name. Marianne went to a local lawyer and filed for a divorce. I understand that Stanley was dumbfounded by it all. He had never had a cross word with Marianne. He couldn't understand the sudden disappearing act (as he called it), until he was served with divorce papers a few days after Marianne disappeared. The fact of the matter was, Marianne wanted Stanley's name! After all, to make it as an actress in Hollywood, Marianne Marks sounded a lot better then Marianne Vermeer-Rhemrev.

    She rented a small apartment in Los Angeles, located near Hamilton High School. The apartment had a tiny kitchen, a small bedroom upstairs with a bathroom, that was also located upstairs. The living room and kitchen were also very tiny but that didn't matter. Marianne was determined to make it no matter what she had to do. The small apartment was just fine with her. She could afford it. Unbelievable as it may seem, Marianne signed a contract with a modeling/talent agency on her first day in Hollywood. This phenomenon wasn't too hard to understand, when one considers, as I have told you throughout this book, that Marianne was a beguiling beauty. A show stopper! Whenever she went into a market or a restaurant or anywhere, for that matter, heads would turn. She was gorgeous, but not pretentious. She was a class act, all the way. Her agent was from Israel, a woman, who herself was a statuesque beauty in her day. She knew that Marianne had that certain something and she was right. Within two short weeks Marianne was in front of the camera, posing for photographs arranged by her agent. Two weeks later, her photograph was on the cover of one of the most popular photographic magazines in the nation.

Marianne was making a name for herself as a photographic model. She was a favorite of Vidal Sassoon, who used her as a Hair model. Ladyfingers used Marianne as their leading Hands model and Marianne s likeness was used on Sweetheart Soap.

Besides modeling her hair and her hands, Marianne had a magnificent body and was sought after by leading magazines. Her agent and Marianne were very selective about who could photograph her, for what products and publications etc., because Marianne had her sights on an acting career. In between her modeling sessions, Marianne was in acting school. She took it seriously and she learned the craft. One day, her agent called and told Marianne that she had arranged a reading for a casting director for a television series program called *Fantasy Island.*

Marianne walked into the casting director s office and walked out with her first co-starring role! She had the magical look of an island princess. The casting director was thrilled. As I have repeatedly said, Marianne was a beguiling beauty. Now the equation was enhanced with acting.

As time went by, Marianne co-starred on many series television programs including, but not limited to; *Fantasy Island, Love Boat, Baretta, Code Red, Chips* and more. She won a co-starring role with Sam Elliot in the ABC Movie, *Wild Times.*

When she read for the famous director Richard Brooks, she was cast in a co-starring role with Sean Connery in the action adventure, *Wrong Is Right.*

In February, 1977, Marianne met me; writer, producer, director, Jerry Schafer. It was love at first sight for both of us. I was raising a four year old son by myself, in my Pacific Palisades home. Marianne came to read for me that afternoon, for a role in a television variety show that I was directing. I hired her, without hearing her read one word! My God, I thought that's the most beautiful woman I have ever seen.

That night, I went home and was going over the list of people I had read that day for the various roles in the show. I came across Marianne's photograph and phone number. What have I got to lose, I thought. I called her and she answered the phone. "This is Jerry Schafer," I said. "Would you go to Knot's Berry Farm with me and my four year old son?"

Without any hesitation, Marianne said, " I'd love to!" Then, she said, "You've got a four year old? I'll bet he's cute, What's his name?" I replied by saying "His name is Aaron." Then she asked, "When do you want to go?" "How about tomorrow?" I replied instantly. Marianne asked what time I wanted to go. "How about 4 o'clock?" Then, I said, "We can pick you up at four. I'd like to take Aaron on a few rides and we can have dinner at the restaurant out there. They say it s great. How does that sound?

Marianne hesitated for a moment. I remember thinking she was going to change her mind, because she remembered an appointment or something but I was wrong, Okay, she said. I ll be ready at 4.

I was thrilled. I told Aaron that tomorrow I was taking him to Knot s Berry Farm and we would go on rides and have dinner. I also told him I was taking a girl with us. Of course, he wanted to know who she was. I told him she was an actress, a beautiful actress, I said.

Is she going to be my Mother? he asked.

Well, I said. I don t know about that, I told him, we ll see.

At exactly four, we pulled up to her apartment complex. I rang the bell. Her voice came over the speaker, Is that you, Mr. Schafer?

Yes it is. Are you ready? I asked.

I ll be right down. she replied. Then, within a few moments, she opened the gate. My God, she was beautiful. She was wearing a yellow outfit that made her radiate. I helped her into the limo. Immediately, Aaron jumped onto her lap. That s how our date began. It was fabulous. We went on rides, ate cotton candy and got to know each other, at least a little. Aaron was the star of the show. Marianne couldn t leave him alone and he wouldn t leave her alone. They held hands most of the time. I guess we seemed like a family taking in the sights and sounds of that fabulous place.

I remember thinking that I never wanted the night

to end. I couldn't believe that Marianne agreed to date me in the first place. Now that we were together, I couldn't believe how natural it all seemed. In a way, it seemed like it was the way it was supposed to be and, as it turned out, it was.

Two years later, on October 1st, 1979, we were married in the Bridal Suite at the Brown Palace Hotel in Denver, Colorado. From the day I met Marianne in 1977 to today as I am writing this book, I have never dated or been with another woman.

During our marriage, Marianne was not only my wife, she became my partner, my lover, my best friend, my everything. She said, "Honey, all I want to do is make it possible for you to be creative. I will handle everything else." And, she did. Through twenty-three years of marriage Marianne and I produced over 175 television programs together. Marianne starred in many of them. Every time I wrote a show, I wrote the leading female role for her. Nepotism be damned, Marianne was right for each thing we did. She was a bundle of talent.

After ten years of marriage, Marianne not only ran our house and every aspect of it, she had learned the production business and became my most valuable asset in that regard too. When I would write something, I would give it to Marianne. She would correct my mistakes, add her creative nuances and more. I used to love to watch her working at the computer. I would watch her eyes and could see her intelligence. I always noticed her posture. Marianne was like a mannequin, sitting perfectly straight in the chair. Yes, Marianne could write, produce and act. She did it all, including, acting as the Operations Director for our companies.

In between her responsibilities in the business world and her never-ending work around our house, Marianne hosted television game shows, talk shows, sporting events, musical variety shows, documentary programs, institutional commercials and, she acted in movies and more. No matter what we did, we did it together. When I would leave the house to go to a meeting, Marianne never failed to call on our cell phone just to tell me that she was thinking about me and that she loved me. For me, it was the same. I couldn't wait to get home to her. When I would walk into the house, I couldn't wait to see her smiling face and kiss her. Sometimes, when we were working on a show, we would spend twenty hours working at home, me in my office area and Marianne in hers. We didn't talk during the day, but we both knew that the other was there and that was all that mattered. I know it seems like I'm writing things about my Marianne that to some people, would seem impossible. Well, let me tell you more. On top of everything else Marianne could do, she was also a fabulous cook. She cooked different dishes for me almost every night. One, was better then the other. I never missed the opportunity to thank her. I was so grateful to be married to her. I felt fortunate to be able to be in her company. I will be thankful to God to my dying day, for giving me Marianne.

Now, without my Marianne, I know that my life will now take a turn that is quite different from what I am used to. I also know that I will never love another woman, as long as I live. I am looking forward to being with my Marianne, when it is my time to go. That is the thought that stays in the front of my mind constantly.

My friends are trying to help me through this period of grieving, but to no avail. I am so sad and broken hearted. I wonder if I will ever be able to be creative again or laugh again or even have an intelligent conversation with anyone again. I know that people cry when they lose a loved one because much of the time, they are crying for themselves. In this respect, I have tried to analyze myself and have decided that isn't the case with me.

I reach over in the morning to take her hand and she's gone. I just miss her. I miss the sound of her voice. The whole package (as they call it) was the most wonderful part of my life. Now it's gone forever. Only the memory is left.

I remember how Marianne ran our companies with an iron fist. Try to over bill International Video Communications, Inc., our television production company or Sanford International, our movie production company and you would have to deal with a very exacting Marianne Marks Schafer.

Marianne was not only beautiful, intelligent and talented, she could charm a king cobra or back down the toughest negotiator. She had the most incredible advance awareness of any person I have ever known.

Through the years of our marriage and business relationship, we traveled much of the world together; Japan, Canada, Holland, Sweden, Belgium and France. As the years passed, we continued producing a variety of programs. We also started putting our USA Series together. To accomplish the logistics, we traveled the 50 states during the development phase. Often, a new person would come into our lives. Marianne could sense danger. "Forget about him," she'd say and that would be that! I had come to realize just how accurate her feelings about people were. She hit the bulls eye every time.

I wrote a movie for Marianne. In between everything else we were doing it was very important to me to write a film that she would star in.

The film was called, *Fists of Steel*. We shot it in Hawaii in 1988. Unfortunately, the business people connected to that project caused the movie to be a financial disaster for us. Not for them, for us! As we were negotiating for the production funds Marianne warned me to be careful of the people we were dealing with. "I don't trust them," she said. At this point in our business, we had exhausted our funds. We had spent a fortune traveling to 775 cities, towns and rural areas of America, locating the areas we wanted to video tape, as part of the USA series. As a result of spending so much, I was desperate. I wanted the finance, no matter what. Because of that desperation, I didn't listen to my Marianne, in spite of what I have told you about her innate sense of people. As a result, the film was stolen from us and we lost millions of dollars, dealing with unscrupulous people from Chicago.

The fact of the matter was, Marianne was outstanding in the film. She was beautiful and acted her role with great intensity and honesty. She was wonderful. The loss of the money was one thing. The loss of the film that we had worked on for a year was another. This had never happened to us before. It was a terrible tragedy for us both.

We had made arrangements with good friends

Angel In My Pocket

throughout the nation, to present our film in a way that would insure great financial success. As it turned out, when the backers got greedy and stole the film, we saw to it that those things didn t happen. It broke Marianne s heart. She never got over it and neither did I. I knew I had to pull the rabbit out of the hat, so to speak, when I started working on an idea to create a mobile post-production unit, that would be interchangeable in all forms of video production.

After a couple of months of working with Sony engineers, I came up with the drawings for the unit. I also came up with the cost of 1.4 million dollars!

When we were in Hawaii making *Fists Of Steel*, I met a fellow who asked me if I would help him, out by putting his wife into our film. Her name is Jeannine, he said. She needs her SAG card, He said, If you will help me, I will appreciate it very much. He smiled and said, By the way, my wife is a marvelous actress, with lots of experience in Europe. The man seemed so sincere and was so respectful to me, that I agreed to use his wife, sight unseen. And, we did use her. She played her part just fine. We were all happy.

During the filming, Marianne met Jeannine and she liked her. In fact, after we finished the film and returned to our home in Las Vegas, Marianne stayed in touch with Jeannine on the telephone. As fate would have it Marianne told Jeannine about our new Project, The Mobile Post-Production Unit. She also told her that we were looking for the finance of 1.4 million dollars to build it. When Marianne told me that she talked to Jeannine about our project, I asked her why. Why would you tell a stranger about our idea," I asked? Marianne looked at me and said, "I just felt like it was a good idea." She smiled at me and I kissed her. Whenever Marianne thinks something is a good idea, it usually is.

A few days later, I received a telephone call from Hawaii. It was the husband of Jeannine. "My wife tells me that you and your wife need some cash to do a project. How much do you need," he asked. I told him we needed 1.4 million dollars to build the first mobile post-production unit in the country. He asked me how much the unit would be worth, when it was completed. I told him if it works, it will be worth more then it's going to cost. I couldn't put a dollar figure to it. He said, "You know something Jerry, I like that answer. Jeannine and I have talked about this. You helped us out when you were here in Hawaii, so I'm going to help you. How soon do you need the money?"

I told him I needed the money as soon as possible, so that I could order the equipment and begin the engineering aspects. "Give me your bank account number," he said. "I'll wire the money tomorrow." I couldn't believe it. Was he really going to send that much money, without an agreement. "What about an agreement? I said. Don't we need an agreement? We can do an agreement later, he said. Just build the unit. If you sell it, I want my money back. If you keep it and it works, pay back the loan any way you can. How about that?" he said. Marianne was sitting next to me during the conversation. She could hear everything that was being said. All she did, was sit there with a big smile on her face. Again, her intuition had paid off. By talking to the wife of this fellow, we received the finance to build our prototype mobile post-production unit. Interestingly, when I agreed to put his wife into our film, I had no idea he was a multi-millionaire.

Marianne worked day and night with me to get the unit built. We ordered equipment from box houses in New York, Chicago and San Francisco. At one point, our house was filled with so many boxes and wires and equipment, that we could barely get through our dining room out to our patio, which was also filled with equipment. Three months later, the unit was completed. It sat in front of our house, waiting to be tested. And test it, we did.

Marianne and I went on location with the unit and video taped a documentary, called *GET MADD*. This turned out to be the most comprehensive documentary ever produced, on the subject of driving under the influence. For her performance that year, Marianne won the New York Television Festival For Best Performance, Best Narration of a Documentary. The program was an enormous success. So was our mobile unit. It worked like a charm. There were a few glitches, but we soon corrected the problems, and went on to produce over forty-five television programs, including a television series using our mobile post-production unit. Marianne and I worked on our America Series in between every show we did. All of the money we earned, went into the America Series. It seemed like a never-ending process, but the production is of gigantic proportions and only two of us were putting it together. Marianne once mentioned to me that if a major motion picture studio had this project, the entire studio production staff and technical crew wouldn t be as far along as we were, even though we had been working on the project for over ten years! I knew she was right. I also knew that no other person, other than Marianne, could have added the creative and insightful things to the project that she brought to it.

As I have repeatedly said, Marianne was incredibly talented and smart. Everything we did connected to this project seemed to work, because we both had the same vision and same purpose. That's the way it was from day one in our relationship.

I am so grateful to God for giving me Marianne and letting me be with her for almost a quarter of a century. I am grateful to God for every single second I got to spend with Marianne; for every word I heard her say, for every time I touched her hand or kissed her beautiful face. I am grateful to God for every time I drove in the car with Marianne or flew on an airplane with her or went shopping with her. I used to love to push the cart and watch her check the list she had made, before we went to a market. Everything was so perfect with her, down to the price of a piece of cheese. If it was on sale, Marianne knew about it and targeted it for our refrigerator. I am grateful to God for being able to say that Marianne is my wife and I will love her until the day I die.

When I first started going with Marianne she told me that cancer ran in her family. Her father and mother both died of the disease. Marianne was certain that she would also get it. I listened to what she said. She said it many times. I knew there was a possibility that this could happen, but Marianne was so health conscious, I didn't believe it would happen to her. She was careful of what she ate, conscious of how she exercised every day and she maintained very strict rules for herself, in this regard. Marianne was aware of what she needed to do to stay healthy. Marianne generated so much 'life' just being around her. It was impossible for me to believe that she would ever be stricken with cancer. Our life together was filled with work. Of that, there is no doubt. We had great enjoyment and satisfaction when a project was completed and another one began. We were together all the time. We were inseparable. That's the way it was. We were never apart, no matter what was going on. Even when I was at the studio, I had my walkie-talkie and Marianne had hers. IVC one to IVC two…her beautiful voice would come over the walkie-talkie. Marianne called me intermittently, throughout the day, every day! We loved each other so much. I have read many love stories. I have produced and directed love stories and I have written love stories. My wish is that every reader of this book will find someone they will fall in love with, like I found my Marianne. Love can be measured by how much time you want to spend with a person. As Ben Franklin said, "Time is the stuff that life is made of." The time you spend together is the most important ingredient for a lasting romance.

I dedicate this book to the loving memory of my wife, Marianne Marks Schafer who I will never stop loving and who I will carry inside of my heart until the day I die.

JERRY SCHAFER

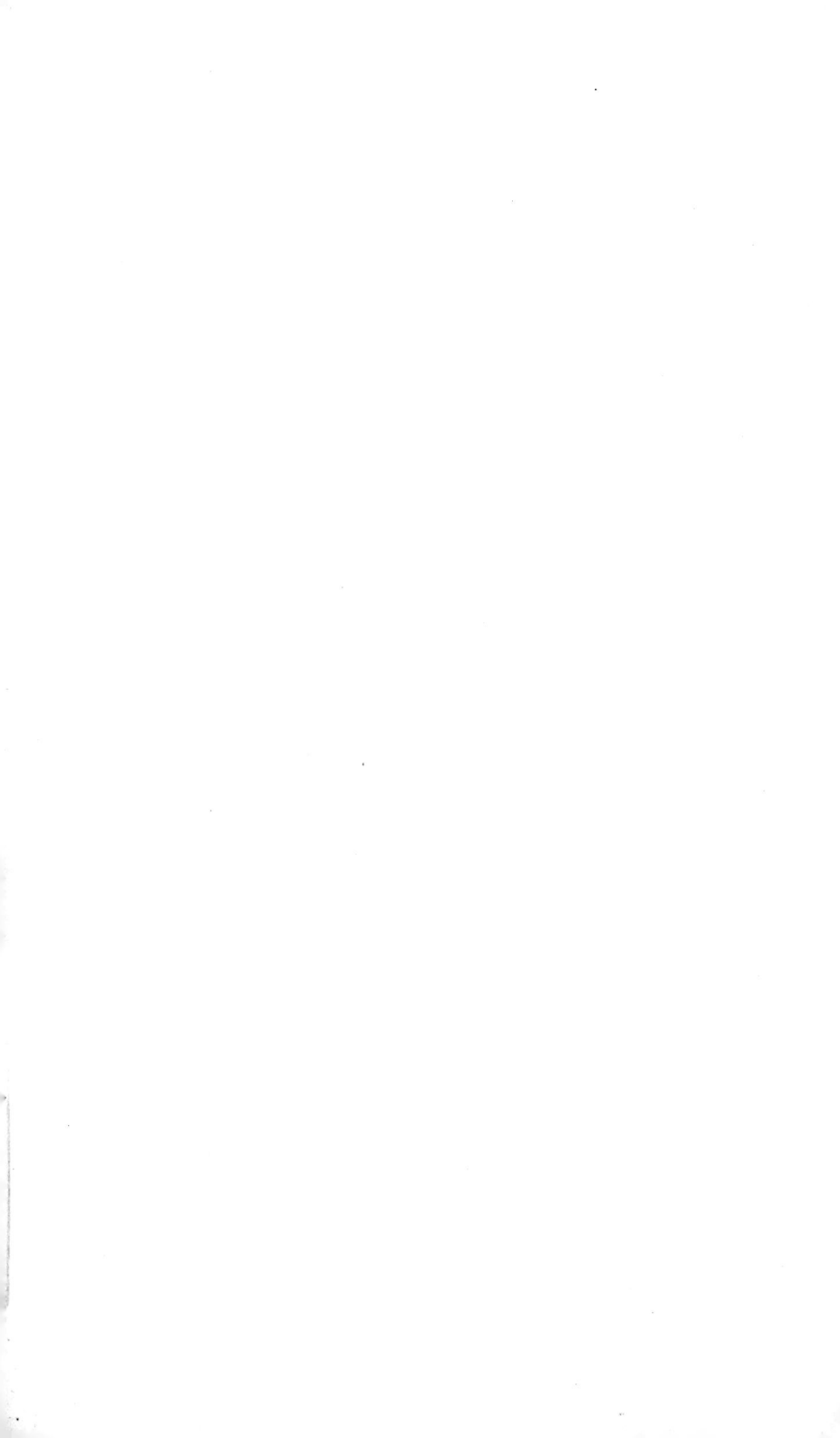